DEDICATION

For my fearless patients and their families who inspire and
teach me daily

AUTHOR'S NOTE:

This book is about celebrating the power of the patient—not the disease or drama. The names are changed, but the joys, sadness, and courage are very real. After 25 years of caring for and about cancer patients, I am inspired to share their very human, inspiring, and compelling moments. Very little here is about the cancers. We all know people experiencing health dramas while attempting to get on with life. So many of these perspectives and events are common. With each story, there are several patients who vividly come to mind, and I relive a similar if not identical event. It is my hope that you will find courage for yourself by spending this time with them as I am blessed to do every day.

LISTENING TO CANCER

The Doctor visits with her truly courageous patients.

"Hi. **Mr. Davis**. How are you doing today?"

"Hey, Doc. I HAVE...CANCER!"

We both burst out laughing, not because cancer by itself is funny, but because of the context. After all, *everyone* I see has cancer, and Mr. Davis, who was receiving treatment for it wanted to surprise me. In that moment, I was the patient and he was the doctor. He gave me an out-loud laugh that carried me through the rest of the morning.

MARY MAE

Mary Mae is always a bundle of taught energy. The high-strung, wild curls on her head seem even more energized when she is talking. "Doc, I have to get back to work. I am working 12-13 hours a day. I don't have time for this breast cancer. I have to support my family. No, I can't get out to counseling even though my husband can't handle the diagnosis and left me."

This went on for months. No time for tiny Miss Curly Head. Everyone and everything else was on the radar, pulling her in every other direction. Then one day it all stopped. The room was painfully quiet. She would not, could not go to work that day. She had become very ill very quickly. In just a few short months, her disease came roaring back and was everywhere. The tiny 40-year-old aged in front of my eyes. Gone was the concern for the job, the house, the husband, the traffic, the work pressures, and the family dynamics. It was just Mary and the terrifying truth. This would be the end of her life. She would get treatment, but the inevitable had arrived. Maybe the frenetic pace over the past year had been hope; maybe it had been an effort to push this possible reality away from focus. It is startling just how focused you become when this somber message gets to the brain. It's a close relationship between no time for me and no time period.

SALLY

"But it IS all about me!" **Sally** blows into the department with the wild, flowing scarf tied around her head. She is not trying to hide the fact that she is bald; instead it is her badge of courage! She is an honest-to-goodness survivor on every front. She has laminated every story printed about her and hangs them in our lady's dressing rooms, hoping to inspire others.

"Look how great I did; look at the trooper I am; look at my courage; look at the stories, some of them pages long; look at what a fighter I am. You can do it too!" Ego and energy. When I come into the room, I see the video of her sanctuary at home her husband lovingly built for her. A garden of hope and healing, a place for reflection. This is her way of dealing with the cards. While I take it all in, I look to her side. I see the loving and supportive husband, the glow in his face. Building both their lives around this drama, his identity now tied with hers on this journey. I think how wonderful it is to have this support. I also wonder how he'll survive when she is gone.

ANNIE

There is a glow. No, it's not in the face or the eyes. It's on a PET scan. It's the radiographic finding of a tumor, of cancer, of the writing on the wall. **Annie** knows this. She's been there before. Cancer is a chronic disease - how chronic and for how long is always the $64,000 question. You would like to reach for an eraser, grab the mouse, put a box around it, and hit delete. The stupid, bright, yellow-orange glow is mocking us. Really, it's just a tiny thing, no bigger than a blueberry. But a 1cm tumor has 1 billion cancer cells. There's no such thing as "a little." It's like being a little pregnant.

She thinks she knows what I am going to say: "Go to chemo; more radiation; the tumor's back."

Instead I give her a hug; her husband takes her hand and sobs. They have only been married seven years. They thought when they found each other late in life that they'd get more than that. They are being cheated by a stupid, glowing blueberry!

I look her in the eyes and say, "Annie, ignore it. If I did not scan you, you would never know it's there. You play tennis, you work, you love, and you enjoy making cupcakes for your grandchildren. I cannot have you stop your life for this."

Maybe it's my own wishful thinking, maybe it's just what she needs to do. I make a deal.

"Put it away and don't think about it. Live your life."

I will take the glowing "blueberry" and worry about it. Then when I am ready we will look at another scan and decide if we are ready to change her life - only when it's worth it. We will never rid ourselves of every cancer cell. We do, however, manage our own cancers every day. Our immune systems help us fight it. Annie needs all the joy she has to help her. Maybe that's why she only has a blueberry, not an entire cantaloupe!

DR. BENNETT

The professor comes through the door like a stereotype: nappy jacket with patch leather elbows, worn cuffs, knit (Yes, knit. I have not seen one in years!) tie, and even longish graying hair and a slightly dramatic, affected speech. I am already guessing: Does he have a lip or tongue cancer from smoking a pipe? What bought him a ticket to the radiation unit? It is all to be revealed sooner rather than later.

As he sits on the exam table, I begin the exam. As I check the cranial nerves in the face and eyes, I see nothing yet. The oral exam: tongue, oropharynx, pharynx, and tonsils are without surprise. Then to the lymph nodes in the face and neck. I move the hair gently from the area by the left ear, and there is the culprit. You would think that there might be a few moments prompting projectile vomiting when you've been doing this for over 20 years. This was one of them! Not only was the entire ear gone, but there were maggots too! How the heck did he live with this mess?

When I composed myself, I asked the obvious question. (No, it was not, "Can you hear out of that thing?!") I turned to his wife and said, "Do you sleep in the same room?"

Because really I could not imagine how she allowed this to go on. The smell was horrid. After all the treatments, when he finally had a clean, cancer free, if still deformed, ear, she admitted her husband had forbidden her to ever speak of the problem, so she had suffered in silence. Intelligence is not a permit for control.

BARBARA

"They're just plastic bags!" **Barbara** is a 50-something post-menopausal woman with a new diagnosis of breast cancer. She is "fed up" with her voluptuous breast implants obtained when she was 40 years old. She tells the story of all the unwanted attention to her breasts over the past few years with multiple mammograms, ultrasounds, biopsies, and ultimately the cancer diagnosis. She states that this is "punishment for vanity." Nothing dissuades her from her self-flagellation.

I have advised her that she can still receive radiation and then renewal of the implant because radiation can cause contracture and deforming. She wants no part of them and has made getting rid of the "jelly-filled balloons" part of her cancer treatment. Barbara has a plan. She's going to visit a lingerie shop and get the "balloons" on the outside this time.

KAREN

36-year-old **Karen** has decided to undergo bilateral mastectomies. Not an easy decision, but with mother, grandmother, aunts, and cousins with breast cancer, her own positive biopsy did not come as a big surprise. Genetic testing was negative, just proving that we only have slivers of information about this complex disease. Obviously we do not have the testing to prove which gene is the culprit for her. Karen cared for her mother until her death from breast cancer at 66. She tells me that she is a late bloomer, has just completed her master's degree, is looking for work in a new city, and is eager to start dating. She can't believe this curve ball just came her way. She is royally pissed off.

After a tearful and trying visit, we both decide there is a hidden benefit to Karen losing her size-D breasts. I ask what she does for fun. She is a runner. Now she says she looks forward to the freedom this will bring to her athletic life, not having those "flapping around." She's planning on implants (small ones) for reconstruction down the line but says maybe she'll enjoy a boyish figure with her bald head and "confuse the hell out of everyone." A sense of humor can't hurt.

RICHARD

"Doc, I have a headache."

When a stressed, 35-year-old woman says this, it might be a migraine. When a 65-year-old retired man does, he gets an MRI. For **Richard**, an ugly looking abnormal mass of grey swirls confirmed the suspicion. A biopsy needle stuck right through the skull into the mass found even uglier, angry cancer cells called Glioblastoma. This is quite an awakening for a man who just moved from snowy Upper Michigan to sunny Florida to retire.

"Ain't that a kick in the head, Doc?"

I'll say. This is one of the most, if not the most, deadly forms of cancer. Life expectancy for an unresectable tumor like Richard's could be six months. His wife has the deer in the headlights look. She supported him through his career, moved here so he could golf year-round. She'll be by his side through the chemo and radiation. She is not prepared for the other part of the discussion. She cannot see herself without him. It's not as if they took time for granted. According to both of them, they enjoyed a rich and full 40 years together. His wife had thought she would have a new Florida life - you don't have to shovel sunshine. They had just settled on the house, and it even had a sparkling pool for when the grandchildren visit! They thought they'd have another 15-20 years. That's the thing about cancer. It does not wait until you are ready to meet it. It always appears uninvited. It is shocking. It is a thief. It changes your world, forever.

MARCY

"The great thing about this treatment is that I can go surfing with my boys this summer!"

She is spunky, athletic, fun, easy-going, a pure delight. **Marcy** is in her young 30s and has two young teenage children. It is June, and they love to surf. Of course mom can tag along because they still need a driver, but I watch their interaction, and I know they all adore each other. The boys are protective, and she is being tough for them - such a common scenario I never tire of watching. Marcy has just finished a grueling course of neoadjuvant chemo. That's when the chemo is given soon after diagnosis but before surgery to shrink the disease. Then bilateral mastectomies—not because she has any family history but because she says, "Why would I ever want to go through this again? I'd rather just get it all done now." Starting radiation releases her from the weeks of debilitating chemo side effects. She'll be fatigued but able to hang out with the boys. By the end of the summer, her hair is spiked with gel. She is tan, happy, and anxious about their going back to school.

"They had the best summer of their lives. I'll miss them so much. It's hard to believe, Doc, but I appreciate having gone through this. Cancer brought us so much closer!"

Who knew!

BENNY

6'5" overflows the length of the hospital bed, but **Benny** is all bones and joints. He lived his life on a shrimp boat, a very common career in this area, but for Benny that life ended with the Gulf oil crisis. After the spill, he lost his living situation on the Gulf and moved in with his brother here. They both noticed a growing lump in his cheek, and I am certain that, if not for his brother, he would not now be at this hospital. The workup and diagnosis found a large mass from melanoma. He probably had a small lesion on his skin that was never seen through the tough, tan-weathered skin but spread to lymph nodes and grew rapidly. Even just a few millimeters of melanoma is dangerous; this looks like a wad of chewing tobacco. It's the only plump thing on his thin, drawn face.

The team convenes and discusses a plan of care. He is only 52 years old. As we are telling him what is going to take place, sometimes completely ignoring that he is under that sheet, he reaches for my arm. He tugs on my sleeve, and all the weariness is evident behind those sunken blue eyes.

"Doc, is it really worth it?"

As the cancer team, we have a complex plan in place, but I don't have an answer for him.

RALPH

"Okay, that's it. I am going to the nunnery!"

Raised Roman Catholic with friends from high school who joined the order, I actually do know what that is. But **Bernice** is a free-spirited, Jewish lady from the Bronx.

"Hugh Hefner at 84 is engaged to a 24-year-old blond bombshell. I am sick of online dating where the men my age and even older just see me as their old, tired, former wife. They want the mid-life dream. These younger women will scoop them up because they don't have to wait and struggle for the lifestyle. It's already there, and the men are so grateful, they get everything!"

Bernice is a fun, bright, beautiful, interesting, and smart lady—lots to offer a relationship if she can find one. That day **Ralph** came in for a follow-up. When patients have radiation treatment, it's every day Monday through Friday for weeks. He always delighted in getting out of the assisted living home where he lived since his wife died eight years ago. We had not seen him for several months since he finished his treatments. He was all dressed up and brought all his 80–year-old Brooklyn charm to the visit.

When I asked how he was doing, he said, "Doc, I am lonely."

I told him that with his energy and personality, he must be a big hit with the ladies where the ratio is about 10 to 1.

He said, "They are all old! They don't bother wearing their glasses, so they can't see how good looking I am. They can't hear my stories because they can't see to find their hearing aids, and the few who can hear don't get my jokes. By the time I am done explaining them, we both have forgotten what I was talking about. One said to wrap it up because I was taking too long and she was getting lost. I can't take it. I need a younger woman to talk to."

Once the exam was over, I called Bernice into the room. I put the two former New Yorkers together, and they chatted and laughed for quite awhile. They both let their personalities sparkle. They entertained each other, and their dopamine and oxytocin levels increased. If you overheard, you would have thought they were 30 years old and on a date.

As Bernice helped to wheel Ralph out to the lobby, he looked up and winked at me saying, "Now that's what I'm talking about!"

I told Bernice she was the doctor today. She smiled and said, "Thanks, I needed that too".

STEVE

In radiation therapy, almost all patients come in with a diagnosis. Many have extensive workups and testing. Too many have had symptoms for a long time before they seek medical care. When I walk into the room, chart in hand, the diagnosis is on the front page. I did not need the chart this time.

Steve, a big, burly, 42-year–old, bearded, gruff man was pacing the room. Not because I was late. I try to be diligent about wait times. My patient's time is very valuable. Cancer is frequently life–shortening, so who am I to waste any precious moments for them? I asked Steve to have a seat so we could talk, but he preferred to stand. He told me that as a long-distance truck driver, he thought it was just hemorrhoids for 18 months of bleeding. When he could not sit, he bought a donut pillow; when the bleeding increased, he tried pads. Finally, he was too weak to drive. He went to the emergency room, and his hemoglobin was 4 (normal is 12–15).

Most patients I see with bleeding have levels in the 7–8 range. This was the most dramatic drop I'd ever seen. He had been compensating for a long time. He'd had six units of blood that night. They essentially had to replace his entire system. Unfortunately, that did not stem the bleeding, so we need to start radiation immediately. I quickly guessed that he did not even get a colonoscopy for the diagnosis and biopsy. When I examined him, the tumor has grown right out of the rectum. Once again, we will have to play catch up.

Frequently, people wait too long, and then we are racing to start therapy in 24 hours. Medical professionals are human too. I've heard someone say,

"Poor decisions on your part are not an emergency on mine." I don't feel that way. I am here to dig in quickly and help.

We rallied the team. We got therapy started that day, but I was worried because radiation does not work that quickly, and he still needed aggressive management and transfusions until we could get some control of this mess. It was too painful for him to be on his back, so we treated him face down. I was dismayed how stoic he has been trying to work to support his family, ignoring his own pain, staying in denial for them. It was too late; he died later that week of a heart attack from the anemia.

DENISE

"I can't be walkin' down no aisle with this thing stickin' out of my neck!"

It's **Denise,** and she has a large mass about the size of a grapefruit (Docs love to describe tumors as food—it humanizes them.). She has Hodgkins Lymphoma. It came on rapidly, grew down into her upper chest, and caused shortness of breath. She is due to be married in six weeks. Her "man" (they are both just 20) is looking like he wants to bolt. We send her off to chemo and expect she will be a beautiful bride since these tumors shrink quickly.

I see her for radiation after six months of chemotherapy. She is with her mother. The groom had been getting more than he bargained for, and he was a no-show at the wedding. Good for her.

4 years later, she is in for follow-up. Denise went back to school after her treatments. She moved home with her parents and had the loving support she needed there. She graduated college and got a master's in art therapy. She is in a new, loving, accepting relationship, is starting her first new job as an art therapist, and can't believe what a positive force cancer was in her life. We are both overwhelmingly proud.

JEFF

Jeff is a macho, 22-year-old construction worker with testicular cancer. He can't believe his family jewels have decreased by 50%. He is with a pretty blond girlfriend, and there is only one thing on their minds. We have to discuss the side effects to treatment of the abdominal lymph nodes like fatigue and nausea, but I can see that he has little patience for the details. I know each patient is at a different point in their lives. Their concerns may be a child they care for, an adult aging parent that needs them, a spouse that is ailing and they need to survive for, the economics of a lost wage earner on the entire family, if they will suffer or be in pain, how they can still remain in their home alone. The number of different concerns equals the number of cases I see. You think that you could guess, but sometimes they still blindside you.

I try to address them right out of the gate and put them at ease or come up with a plan. I think I know the questions here: Can I be sexually active? Will I be radioactive? Can I still have children? Nope. The burning question: "Can she catch this from me?" How very sweet.

I smile and say, "No, I can say with 100% certainty, your girlfriend will not ever get testicular cancer."

FRED

Fred is 62. He is African American. This is important because prostate cancer frequently occurs younger and more aggressively in this population. He is with a very angry wife. She sits with her arms crossed and won't say a word. Her posture says it all. After the exam and discussion about radiation, an excellent choice for prostate cancer, I send her out to the front desk to set up an appointment which will give me a few moments alone with the patient.

Fred says, "Doc, you gotta help me. I can't even live with her. She thinks if I have prostate cancer, that means I cheated on her. No matter what I say, she won't believe I've been faithful, and I'm tellin' the truth. What can I do? Now I have to battle the cancer and her, too."

Fred and his wife need counseling; they need to talk; they need to focus on the problem and treatment. Prostate cancer may affect 80% of men by the time they are 80 and many will not need any treatment, but it is a different disease in younger men and black men, and it is still the second leading cause of death in men in general. Now I ask Fred to have a seat in the waiting room, and I call his wife back to talk about prostate cancer. We discuss that Fred did not get this by indiscretions and that it is the most common cancer in men.

She starts to listen, but there is no dramatic changing of the mind today. As Fred comes in for treatment (44 days), I watch them together. She becomes more attentive; they touch hands; she smiles; there appears to be relief; she is opening up, and he makes her laugh. By the end of the treatment, they are planning a trip. They have reconnected through the process, and I am happy for them. It could have gone either way.

PHYLLIS

Phyllis is sitting in the "head and neck" exam chair and just about spitting nails. She has a gruff, hoarse voice that would be considered deep and sexy if she were not here in a cancer center. Her "expensive salon" hair, the designer bag and shoes, and the exquisitely tailored suit all cannot distract from the knitted, pinched facial expression. Botox will not change this; only acceptance will. She is far from ready for that. She has blame and is not shy about expressing it. She is in this predicament because she has HPV positive throat cancer. "Thanks to my good-for-nothing, former husband. Can you believe I nurse him through a heart attack, and he finds another woman? I divorce him after 43 years together, and get this in the settlement."

There is no placating her that the virus is ubiquitous and not a direct "insult" from her husband. Her stress over the past year caused a 40 lb weight loss, and now she has anorexia. This is a real problem going into treatment because it is very toxic therapy to the head and neck area, and she will require chemo as well. I thread the nasopharyngoscope through her nose and down her throat to look at the tumor. It is large and hindering movement of the vocal cords, hence the hoarseness.

Phyllis works at her job every day through therapy. She needs the income now. She has more internal fortitude than she ever knew. After seven long weeks of chemo and radiation, she has lost more weight, refusing to have a feeding tube. She is tired, hoarse, and generally weary. We complete the treatment on time, and she never missed a day of work. She is what we call a "trooper" and becomes an inspiration to other patients and staff.

When Phyllis comes back for follow-up months later, the tumor is gone; the PET scan is negative. She has a new apartment and a promotion; she is back in her designer clothes, bright and cheerful. She sits primly in the head and neck chair.

I say, "You look maaaarvelous!"

She says, "I had Botox!"

Pop-Pop

It's often not about the cancer. The diagnosis incites fear and trepidation even in the lionhearted. So often, patients fear the life changes it demands. Many patients tell me they did not plan on this, and I often say that cancer is very inconvenient. That is a gentle way of saying, "Pay attention. This is important." One of the reasons I love my work is that I have the privilege of helping people at a critical time in their life. Cancer affects every aspect of a person's life. This is an incredibly courageous group; there are over 12 million cancer survivors. We all know someone who is one. Their words live with me.

Like Mary, a lay religious with breast cancer who said, "Do whatever you need; I am going to live until I die and no longer!"

Like Reverend Tom, so fearful of the diagnosis of metastatic disease, who said, "Doc, am I going to die?" and I said, " Reverend, we all will, but why don't you let that go and live now?"

Like Thelma who smiled: "Cancer may have beaten my body, but it saved my soul."

There is Gene, the homeless man, who just loved coming in here to the waiting room, eating cookies, and watching TV. (If only we had a shower!)

Then there is Nathan, whose mother was being treated for extensive cancer. They lived in a shelter and she would not survive. The folks in the waiting room took up a collection for them and gifted Nathan toys for Christmas.

It's intimidating to go through all of this. You would think you could get to be old without the insult. Jack's little great-granddaughter, who is two, comes with his daughter who babysits her. She is the sandwich generation. He is confused and has dementia, so there is a lot going on when they arrive each day for treatment for his skin cancer. Her **Pop Pop** asks over and over, again and again, "What are we doing here? Where are we?"

Finally, Annalise, the great-granddaughter, has had enough. She pops the binky out of her mouth when his daughter was too weary to respond for the 15th time and says, "Pop Pop, we are at the Radiation Unit, and you are going to get radiated!"

Finished, she sticks the binky back in. The two-year-old is now in control.

MARGIE

Margie needed a mammogram. She had endometrial (uterine) cancer five years ago, and there is a relationship between these hormone sensitive cancers. When I set her up for the scan, she said "I am not having it for another year because Medicare only pays every other year" (that was true several years ago).

As cancer physicians, we lobbied to get that changed. We realize there is cost to the government, but mammograms may miss a small tumor especially in dense breasts, and then it may be four years between a truly negative study, the one that misses it, and the next one that detects the disease. Although breast cancer is usually not that fast-growing, it could make the difference in a patient being able to avoid chemotherapy.

As I said to Margie back then: "Medicare does not get cancer, people do. You would pay for jeans or for pet food. Why will people accept only the healthcare that is 100% paid for by insurance?" (A screening mammogram at that time was $60).

In most cases, the mammogram would have been normal. In Margie's case, wouldn't you know, she was found to have a 3mm (tiny) ductal carcinoma in-situ—the earliest form of cancer. Easily treated and worth the $60.

CHUCK

Chuck came in for a follow-up after having surgery and then chemo and radiation for lung cancer. This tumor bears close watching since it is the leading cause of cancer death in men and women. The two-year overall survival remains low in spite of aggressive management. Chuck had stopped smoking at the time, but came in more short of breath 18 months later. We checked his scans. Pet CT's are wonderful studies since they reveal not only anatomy but activity. The mass in his chest was still there on CT but showed no activity of cancer cells at all on the PET part of the scan. That was great news. He was seen by a pulmonologist and put on several inhalers. He did not qualify for oxygen since his level was still over 95% on room air.

When Chuck and his wife came in to review the scans, we could see the problem both on him and the scan. He had gained 40 lbs since therapy. The scan showed minimal fat under the skin (the fat that is normally removed by liposuction), but the dangerous fat we all hear about that encases abdominal organs had increased dramatically. The lungs could not expand as the diaphragm could not compress downward into the abdomen, a form of restrictive lung disease. I had a new prescription for Chuck—not chemo or radiation, but exercise. He was to walk 30 minutes twice a day (better than 1 hour at a time to divide it up for maximum benefit). This would not only help to lose the constricting abdominal fat, but also act as pulmonary rehab by requiring chest expansion. It was a win-win for his heart, his lungs, and his wife, who loved a walk on the beach!

CLAY

Clay (I love Southern names) was sent for treatment for a difficult problem. He had lung cancer in the past and now was found to have metastatic disease in the brain. The lung cancer was gone everywhere else, but most chemo cannot penetrate the blood-brain barrier. Therefore, tumor cells carried there through the blood stream can "set up shop" in the brain. This requires radiation. Now we try to treat these tumors with small, local fields, but this occurred when the standard would be to treat the entire brain for ten treatments since he had at least six tumors. The brain radiation would cause hair loss, which could last for several months before re-growing, short term memory loss, hearing loss, possibly cataracts and fatigue. Clay was a vibrant man, very proud and energetic. When I reviewed the scans, I then discussed the side effects for treatment.

He said in his slow southern drawl, "Now, Doc, this here's my problem. I doubt that I am going to beat this thing again, and it looks mighty serious from where I sit. Now I'm tryin' to see myself at my funeral, and you know it's going to be a big one! So here's the deal: I am not going to get this treatment and I am going to die with this disease, but at least I will not lose my hair and I will look good at my funeral. It may sound vain, but it's the last time everyone's going to see me."

I was dismayed, but there was no changing his mind. He was not giving up his looks for the promise of a few more months. Five months later, everyone said how great he looked at the funeral.

HARRY

"What's this treatment going to do to my sex life?"

Not a surprising question since radiation and all treatments for prostate cancer can decrease sexual function over time. **Harry's** question is a surprise as it comes from the 88-year-old curmudgeon sitting on the exam table.

"Look I don't have much time left, and I have to live the most while I can."

I had no objection to this, but being a fairly new practitioner, I had not yet come to grips with not treating. It's much harder to decide to "do nothing" than to come up with a plan to treat. I took this octogenarian and treated his prostate cancer, and in one year at 89 he was impotent. Big mistake. He rightfully was angry, but this lesson was great for all the patients who would follow him in my practice. Listen; treat the patient according to his wishes. Recognize that eradicating the cancer is not the end all. It helped me see the big picture and try to look at all perspectives. I relearn this almost every day. Finding out what is important to the patient and their loved ones and then guiding them to fulfill their wishes—this really turns the table in healthcare. Today, with new guidelines, we wouldn't even think of checking Harry's prostate let alone giving him treatment. At 89, we surely did not extend his life.

ROBERT

The gentleman appeared small and shrunken, almost disappearing in the large hospital bed. He was very ill, and I was consulted to consider radiating his lung to try to relieve the obstruction causing repeat pneumonias. Most patients die from complications from their disease, not the tumor directly. Pneumonia is common. Pulmonary embolism (blood clot), cardiac arrhythmias, and overwhelming sepsis (infection) are all end-of-life events for cancer patients. This man, **Robert**, was ready to rest. He'd had enough. His son was by his bedside. I thought I'd be having discussions regarding treatment. He surprised me with a request.

"We all know that my father is dying. He does not have good insurance. If you do a lot of treatment, we may lose the little assets he has—his house, which we all need to live in, money, which we need to bury him and pay his debts. Please help us not incur more financial burden for just a few more weeks of life. It is not what he would want, and we are in dire need."

I had never been asked that before. We sent the patient to hospice as per his wishes and the family's, and he died two weeks later. Since then I have had this discussion many times with other families. "Do no harm" is more than a physical directive.

MARILYN

Marilyn hobbled in using a fairly useless cane for her follow-up visit. She had been treated for breast cancer two years before. On the hormone therapy, she gained weight, and progressive inactivity and depression resulted in the 315 lbs she now wore sadly on her 5'4" frame. The weight took its toll on her hips, knees, and ankles. She was essentially crippled. She was only 52 years old and a nurse but was now on disability, not from the cancer, but from the weight and joint problems. After I had our medical assistant help me bring her down from the table into a chair with great effort on the patient's part, I rolled up to face her sitting on my stool.

Knees to knees we sat. I put my hand on her leg and said that this had to stop. "I want you to go for gastric bypass surgery. This weight is killing you."

It was 2003, and only highly selected patients were candidates. Her primary care doctor had told her she would not clear her for surgery because of the risk to her heart. I told her she was already dying. What did she have to lose? I told her to either find a new primary care doc or go to the bariatric center and let them decide.

She wept and had great ambivalence. She said she knew she would be dead if she did not do something dramatic. A year later, we closed that office and advised patients to see me in our new hospital facility 25 miles away or return to their medical oncologist for routine follow-up care. On a busy morning in my clinic 18 months later, a beautiful, normal weight, fit woman came in for follow-up. I could not for the life of me place her.

As I came into the room, she jumped off the table and grabbed me in a hug. She said, "Doc, you saved my life!"

It still took me several minutes to get it. I was shocked to see Marilyn and double-checked the name on the chart. This woman had been reborn. She'd had the gastric bypass, now weighed 140 lbs, exercised every day, and had gone back to work as a nursing supervisor. She had new hair color, great jeans, energy, and vitality that all flabbergasted me. We were so excited together and spent an hour catching up. To this day, she remains an inspiration because I hold her story in my heart and encourage others with her strength. We only get one life. Why live it as a victim, whatever the circumstances? It takes courage. Like Marilyn, we just need to find those who will be our champions.

ANDREW

Just because we try to practice the dictum to "do no harm" does not mean we can see the future. So we do the best we can with our current knowledge. I was absolutely convinced that I had the right plan of care for **Andrew**. He presented at 77 years old with widely metastatic prostate cancer. He had what is called a "super scan." The bone scan took up all the Technetium 99 diffusely so that at first sight it looked negative, but on further review, it meant that every bone was diffusely involved with tumor. His PSA was over 2000, and normal is 4ng/ml. (PSA is a prostate specific antigen which is a protein that should only be present in the prostate and circulating only minutely in the blood stream. When it is high, there is something going on in the prostate allowing it to leak out, and in this case other tumors in the body were also contributing to the level.). He had back pain, which was the reason he had sought medical attention. Patients rarely come to the doctors because they have cancer; they usually come in when they cannot manage other symptoms, especially pain.

MRI's confirmed that the bones were diffusely involved. The first plan of care was to reduce the testosterone which was feeding this tumor like fertilizer. Whenever I take a history for prostate cancer, I ask if the patient is sexually active, an important issue because we frequently find that their sexual function has diminished over a few years and may be related to the cancer. The prostate gland has one function and that is to provide fluid to carry sperm from the testicles. A prostate filled with tumor, or a large, even benign prostate, often cannot perform its job, and often the gland compresses the urethra which comes from the bladder directly through the prostate. If there is growth, the prostate can squeeze the urethra, acting like a tight bottleneck. Younger men can "pee like a racehorse;" older men not so much.

Andrew was present with his wife of six years. She blushed when I asked the question, but Andrew was proud and delighted to answer, "We have sex three times a day every day. Retirement is great!"

I looked over at his wife, and she nodded. His testosterone level must be sky high just like his PSA! This was going to be a tough sell to bring this man's testosterone down. This was his lifestyle, and I was about to rip it from him. We had several discussions over the next few weeks. As soon as I would put him on the anti-testosterone hormones, he would be impotent, definitely not his life choice.

Well, unfortunately, the pain increased. He did receive radiation to some areas, in an effort to only palliate but without the hormones. A few months later, it came roaring back, and I really needed to push the hormone issue. He poorly tolerated pain medications (and we tried them all). Ultimately, he reluctantly decided, with the insistence of his wife, that she would rather have him here and more comfortable than lose him. We started the hormone therapy—first an oral dose and then monthly injections. I was rightfully concerned about his tolerance.

His reaction to the hormones was the fiercest I had ever seen. He required hospitalization. It was a noxious stimulus. He had projectile vomiting, more pain, drenching sweats, palpitations, etc. It was horrific for him and his wife and his doctors to witness. I thought he would get used to it after several weeks, but the symptoms were unremitting. Now not only was he not sexually active, but he was in abject misery. This happens; we treat the disease and not the patient. Andrew would have been happier without treatment, lesson learned.

CHARLIE

There is always an interesting dynamic when an entire family accompanies a patient into the office. Just like the general consensus is that time remaining is inversely proportional to the number of IV bags and equipment at the hospital bed side, when my staff is pulling more and more chairs and there is standing room only, the patient's part in the decision making is inversely lessened. Usually I have to hunt through all the introductions to find the, usually, small, frail, elderly patient. Many times the family has convened from several states. I wonder if they are together for the holidays.

There is a positive to this much attention; the doctor will be spending more time with this visit, answering all the questions, trying to figure out the dynamic, and then getting to what the patient wants. I am a big fan of patient advocates. I believe that an extra set of eyes and ears and rational thinking contribute to the best decisions and understanding. The patient is frequently overwhelmed or in pain or frightened, so it's good to have others share the information. Sometimes it's just awful. Period. It's siblings jockeying for position, finger pointing, bullying the patient, martyrdom; there is sometimes concern regarding money or lack thereof; sometimes the primary caretaker is exhausted and begging for help; there are lifestyle changes that may be happening, with the patient moving into someone's home; there are nursing home decisions, transportation for daily visits, the managing of nutrition, medications, learning how to give tube feedings, insulin, paying for medications, juggling children in the home, missing soccer games and vacations, losing jobs and income in spite of family leave, lack of privacy for couples, long-standing in-law issues affecting the dynamic with the couple or patient; occasionally it is the in-law spouse left with all the responsibility. It is tough. It will affect every aspect of trying to care for this patient.

Treating the cancer for **Charlie** meant treating the patient as well as the family. There would be outbreaks of battles right in the exam room, although I never had to call security. Through it all, I recognized one basic commonality: It was grief. Grief for the patient and what it is doing to the family. Grief for each member now personally affected. They were all losing a part of their lives. It was emotionally charged change. I knew they were all grieving, and not just for the patient. I worked to rein it all in and focus. I could only give the answers that best manage the patient. The rest they will have to figure out.

In the end, I was grateful that Charlie had so many who cared—even if for some it was selfish. At least he was not alone.

And then the times come when these situations profoundly move me: The daughter who lovingly adjusts the father's collar; the son who weeps quietly; the grandchild climbing on the lap demanding attention; the prodigal child making amends at the end; the former spouse fulfilling a duty; the niece, now the only living relative, or a friend because everyone else abandoned them; the brother long apart; the grandmother who lovingly raised them; the significant other who the family ignores; the sister pursuing her career who now stops to hold the hand; the father who is once again the tower of strength; the mother who wishes she could take their place.

Can you just imagine the emotions? Surely we have lived many of them ourselves and been that person at one time or another. It is the human factor. It is not science or treatment or decisions. I am humbled to witness these connections. I am moved by every one of them. The physics, radiobiology, science, and medicine quiets, and the miracle of these connections is what heals.

TIM

Tim is a former CEO of a large financial institution. It has nothing to do with his cancer management, and I don't know this when we meet. He is a big man in a small, demoralizing hospital gown. His face is filled with fear, and his eyes are moist. He has just been diagnosed with lymphoma. To a man who had the world by the tail, it's an insult, occurring just months after retirement.

I think to myself, "This is another 65-year-old who thought they were immune or at least had another 15–20 years." That's the thing about cancer; it does not know your time line. It never waits until you are ready. It creeps up like a thief, changing everything.

I introduce myself, and right after we shake hands, he reaches to a small photo by his bedside.

He says, "Doc, this is my grandson. He was born premature, and he is battling for his life. I need to be well for him and my daughter. It is not about me. I must be here to help him through this, and nothing else matters to me. I am not bargaining for my life. He needs me."

As the mother of a profoundly premature infant myself, I understand immediately. We discuss, and I share this with him. He is grateful that I "get it." He is encouraged to know that my own son is 28 now and there is great hope for his tiny one. We get on with the decisions and plan regarding treatment.

Every time I see him, we check in about the baby's progress. There are setbacks for both of them. Grand-pop and baby are almost on a parallel course.

Two years later, when Tim came in for follow-up, he proudly brought his little grandson. He certainly seemed like a normal "terrible two," and I was thrilled, but I know that not one moment, movement, utterance, expression, or tiny squeeze of the hand would ever be taken for granted by Tim. He beamed.

He said, "Thanks for keeping me here, Doc. I am so grateful."

I answered, "No; this sweet child did all that and more."

I am reminded once again that everyone has a reason for living. It may be: "Until my daughter gets married," "Until my grandchild is born," "Until my son comes home from the military," "Until my grandson graduates," or "Until my husband has open heart surgery." This list is long and always inspirational. Very rarely it is for themselves.

DON

He was 79 years old, and had just lost his wife one month prior to pancreatic cancer. They were a loving couple and had celebrated their 60th anniversary. He devotedly cared for her, and they were a true delight to have in the department. I received the call that he had been diagnosed with metastatic cancer, and I thought the message was about the wrong person. When he arrived, he had great pain and admitted he was dealing with this but had not gotten help while his wife was alive. There are many stories about spouses dying within months of each other, more frequently the husband soon after his wife. This would be one of them.

We worked on **Don** with chemo and radiation, but it was really too late. During the treatment, he had something serious to discuss. He and his wife had rescued a darling puppy five years before. He was a source of enormous comfort to Don after his wife died. Now he had only one overwhelming concern: What would happen with Scooter? How could he leave him behind? His daughter did not want the large German shepherd, and he'd had no luck adopting him online or in the paper. It was becoming an urgent issue.

As serendipity would have it, another treating physician asked me how Don was doing, and I said that he really wants it to be over but is holding on for Scooter. A staff member in his office had just told the doc that she was looking to add to her household of other rescue dogs. We put them together, frisky Scooter had a new loving family, and Don went "home" within the week to be with his wife. Amazing!

MARTHA

Martha was a frail senior lady with breast cancer. Her case was straightforward and simple to manage. That was not her drama. She came with her daughter, and there seemed to be more going on than the "garden variety" visit. After we reviewed all the details, I asked what else I could do for them.

She quietly said, "Pray for us."

I pulled up my little stool and waited for them to continue.

She said that she was very worried about her grandson. He had been drinking at a party with friends in college. He had fallen down stairs, and at first his friends thought he was just drunk. Sometime later they realized that he was not just drunk but could not move. He now had paralysis. Martha found a place to discuss her tragic heartbreak while she was coming here throughout the course of her therapy with us. She regularly discussed progress and setbacks. She did not have to suffer in silence but felt free to share in a safe place. Sometimes an interested bystander, perhaps in a doctor's waiting room, could help you say the terrible words out loud and in sharing give you a moment of peace. When Martha came for her three month follow-up, we hugged and I asked how she was. Her beautiful young darling Grandson had died just before Christmas.

"My cancer and treatment is so trivial compared with the rest of life."

I had to agree.

SONA

Sometimes you know cancer by the smell. Unfortunately, it stinks, literally. As you walk in the room, it hits you, and yet as a physician, we are immune, right? The sweet middle-aged lady with the heavy accent was primly seated with a hospital gown on the exam table. She was unable to hide the large mass expanding her breast The breast cancer has invaded the skin, making this the highly-aggressive and rapidly metastatic diagnosis of inflammatory breast cancer. It is a nightmare. She stated that the symptoms had only been present for a few months. She blamed her leg pain and inability to ambulate without crutches on a fall, but instead we could clearly see the bone metastasis on the scans. The cancer was eating away normal bone, leaving her with porous, fragile hips at risk of fracture.

She did not have insurance, which had further delayed her rescue from this devastation. Her husband was speaking a foreign language into his cell phone. Doctors usually frown on this cell phone intrusion, but his big, frightened eyes convinced me he needed this contact for reassurance. Many times it is the patient who is strong, and the spouse falls apart and needs significant help. It's not just the details of office visits, tests, plans, and medications to manage. Often it's the strength and support that we as physicians can give to the family. He needed some confidence that he can pass this drama off to us. I will tell relatives, "You be the daughter or husband or wife; let us handle the rest."

In that poor case, she needed care quickly—that day. We marshaled our forces in various offices at the cancer center and admitted her to the hospital for antibiotics, wound care, and chemotherapy. Without aggressive treatment, she would only live a few months—this was the deadliest of breast cancers.

They barely had time to process or grieve that this "breast infection" was a cancer spreading rapidly through her body and killing her. We had to carry them through the process. They both realized everything else in their life was on hold.

Cancer is like that; it's like a funeral. Life stops for those involved. Nothing is as important. Everything is in slow motion. **Sona** realized that in her native country, nothing would have been done. She would have died quickly of this tumor without treatment. She had come here for the American dream, and now American healthcare was trying to give her and her family that chance.

It makes me proud to be part of a system that takes care of patients like her no matter what her circumstances. I think we love rescuing people in America.

CARL LEE

He's tall, skinny, lanky, black, and very Southern, a real gentleman who stands when I enter the room. His wide smile is toothless, and he is a hoot. He tells stories of driving a truck in 48 states and that he worked for 40 years to give his daughter a better life. He plays the lottery so that if he wins he can travel to see Alaska and Hawaii so he can say he's been in all 50 states. **Carl** always says he's fine no matter what the problem. He has seen, felt, managed, and lived through tough times. He's had to sleep on the road in ice storms, drive all night in the wind-swept rain, and make deadlines; nothing was too much work or effort. He is a man of steel.

Finally when he retired, he was found to have cancer. ("No rest for the weary, Doc.") He wears his loose jeans with a long belt with extra holes drilled because he has become so thin. He smiles like he did just win the lottery. He is a joy to care for and an inspiration. You don't need much to be happy, and he is living proof. It's refreshing to see someone with a relaxed attitude. He's not battling this disease like he has to wring every hour out of life; he is just living the day in front of him.

I'd like to take a lesson, but I can't do it. I am chronically thinking and planning ahead. I think responsibility makes me this way, but here was someone showing me another option. I probably won't change today, but I'll think about it.

KATE

I am not sure if this is mania. The young, 40ish patient looks 25, and she and her girlfriend with her are all giggles. I mean hysterical laughter, and the giggling starts as soon they tumble into the door and lasts through the entire exam. Actually it's annoying, and we watch them in utter dismay. One is the patient with cancer. It has not spread and it is still "fixable." I do not like the c word (cured) because cancer is such a sneaky devil and can reappear when least expected years after patients have been sent on their way "cured," so I like to use "control."

In this case, it's one of those HPV-positive tumors. **Kate** will have to "go through the fire" to be controlled, but today she seems ready for anything and completely unafraid—or is this a defense mechanism? It could be, but why is her friend so hyper too? After going through the scans and serious discussion, she has held it in as long as possible. She looks right at me and bursts out laughing.

I finally give up and laugh with her. I say, "You keep that attitude; I'll worry about the cancer."

We work for two months through that process. She has great success, and I can't help but wonder how much the belly laughing (which she did plenty of daily) improved her immune system and helped. It certainly raised the excitement in the department. Just imagine the elderly men watching these two giggling young women come in each day. I think their immune systems improved as well.

Many patients in the waiting room would say, "I'll have whatever they're having!"

Susie

Several years ago, the health information privacy laws were enacted, and they make it nearly impossible for medical offices to care for patients. But they do have a benefit of keeping your health information from prying eyes. Unfortunately, there are many leaks, and information can still get out. We have exceptions to this law when we discuss patients at a multidisciplinary meeting called Tumor Conference. I chaired many of these over the years, and it's a way for physicians to discuss a plan of care for patients newly diagnosed with cancer without the patient seeing each for an opinion. It hopefully brings many minds into the decision-making so that, when the doctor sees the patient, they have many opinions and greater insight into the care recommended.

At one of these conferences, I was surprised to have one of my friends on the agenda. It was difficult at first to see the woman whom I had known for over ten years trembling on my exam table. Her eyes were as big as saucers and her beautiful face, long, red hair, and gorgeous figure could not hide the terror. Her husband stood by her side as if to physically battle the cancer if it got too close. When I entered the room, I just reached out. She fell into my arms, and we hugged and hugged. She sobbed almost uncontrollably. I took her by the shoulders, and we were eye to eye.

I said, "**Susie,** you will be okay. I promise."

A loud, swooshing gasp escaped her lips. Her shoulders relaxed, and she said, "My daughters…"

I said, "You will live for them, and you will survive."

She said that was all she needed to know. It took a lot of work: bilateral mastectomies, hysterectomy, chemo, and radiation, but a year later, with her dear husband, her advocate through it all, she came in for her follow-up.

She said, "I have something to say to you, Joanne. I knew I was in trouble, and I was terrified, but what you did for me that first day made every bit of pain worth it. You gave me confidence and strength. You understood immediately what I needed, and you were there for me. I cannot thank you enough."

It is now 15 years later. The girls are in high school; Susie has a new house and has moved past being a patient. I will never forget her courage and her words to me. I will always remember when I walk into that room for the first time to put myself in that patient's position. Be honest but never take away hope. Remember that we do not know everything and no patient comes in with an expiration date stamped on their forehead. If they have reason to and want to fight, be their champion. Susie remains a great lesson to me. I am grateful that we went through that together.

VICKIE'S HUSBAND

Sometimes patients' families return for visits after the patient has passed on. They experienced the treatment, held the patient's hand, met weekly with me, and really feel that this has been a part of their life and returning is necessary for their healing. When Vickie came in with a large basket of her husband's favorite snacks (quite a good idea), the staff was very moved by the gesture.

It is these meetings and conversations that are as important as that very first encounter. Perhaps some docs would like to avoid this. It is usually an emotional visit. I find these times enriching and healing for me as well. **Vickie's husband** was treated for metastatic prostate cancer. He lived as many men do, for years with this diagnosis—first thought to just be arthritis until the pain in the bones became too great to manage for even a stoic man. He finally then sought medical attention. After his last hospitalization, he was placed in hospice, a wonderful program when families need the extra help with medications and pain management.

Vickie described his last days and how he waited until his children came in from all over the country and then how he wanted her to leave so that he could die on his own. She wept and smiled and laughed through the telling. It was a joy to know that she had closure. He asked her to take his ashes out on a fishing vessel since he was an avid fisherman, and she was thrilled to do his last bidding—caring for him throughout.

It is really a blessing for spouses to be able to carry out the wishes and make the preparation less painful. It's something I highly recommend— preparation for all of us. Our loved ones should know our wishes. How aggressive do you want to be? What is your living (and dying) will? It's one of the most important discussions to have, and I recommend not procrastinating and getting it in writing. Your family doctor should have living will papers, or you can find them on line. We may not know when, but we may as well take part in the planning. Vickie was happy and content to have direction from her stoic husband.

SHEILA

The 32-year-old girl with the peaches and cream complexion just glowed. "Doc, I can't get that scan done now because I am pregnant!"

"Yeah," I said. "The heck with the scan. Sometimes looking for tumors is just voyeurism."

Sheila had Hodgkin's disease, most common in the late teens and early20s. She's been through several rounds of heavy chemotherapy and radiation. She is due for follow-up studies, but we do not put pregnant patients through the radiation of scans unless it is imperative.

I had a discussion with Sheila and her husband. I said, "You are carrying a new life, and this is a blessing after everything you've been through. You deserve the chance to put this behind you. If the pregnancy is successful, then we can scan afterward and manage any problems then. Let's try to have this baby and not be a patient but a new mother."

Sheila and her husband are visibly relieved. It's so very important to let people live. Sometimes in a cancer center, it's not all about the cancer. As difficult and challenging as battling cancer is, isn't the whole point of treatment about living? What's the sense in fighting if life's not worth living? Sheila will go on to have a family, and the disease will remain in the rear view mirror, a distant memory of a time that hope was fragile, future uncertain, and motherhood unlikely. What a joyful blessing this is today.

TESS

Tess lives to tease the docs. She flirts with the men and compliments the women. Whenever I ask her how she is doing, she answers, "Everyone I can!"

She is incorrigible. I know she is just having fun with us, and we are her entertainment for the day. Sometimes these visits really do make the day for patients, and living alone at 85 years, she's so happy to put her broach and earrings on and have a place to go. So we always appreciate her fun ways and girlish quips.

Today she compliments me on a scarf and says, "That will be a quarter!"

I reply, "Oh no, Tess there is inflation, and the price of compliments went up. Don't you know you have to ask for a dollar? Don't sell yourself so cheap!" So, in the spirit of her fun, I get a dollar out of my purse and give it to her.

She pulls me down to her 4'11 frame and gets very serious and whispers, "Please dear, give this to someone who needs it. I am a multimillionaire!"

So I take my scarf off and tie it to her wheelchair. I say, "Now when you go out with the other seniors, you'll know which chair is yours!"

She leaves with a smile like the cat that ate the canary.

STEPHANIE

After seeing so many patients with really dire problems and nearing end of life, sometimes the real fortitude is needed working with someone with a truly curable disease. **Stephanie** is putting me through my paces and testing whatever patience is left on this day. She has a totally curable disease, and as I have said, I almost never used that "C" word. I believe cancer is contained in most cases, not cured. This tumor in Stephanie, ductal carcinoma in-situ of the breast, is greater than 95% curable in most cases with lumpectomy and radiation and 100% with mastectomy.

She will not accept this. She is convinced she is going to die from this and has hypersensitivity to every aspect of care. We discuss the side effects to treatment, and although as docs we have to describe everything that can happen, most never do. Not in this case; she is convinced that she will have every possible problem. I am weary just thinking about these weekly interactions. I am trying to remind myself that if you are in pain, it does not matter that someone else has greater, terrific pain; yours is 100% to you, not lessened by knowledge of someone else. The same is true for so many aspects of life: money, sadness, grief, fear. If you have a feeling, you are 100% into it.

And so, with cancer, the fact that others (even those around you in the waiting room) have more dire situations does not lessen your fear. It is my responsibility to put the reality to their disease status and give the best information to them. We are not all that altruistic or compassionate or empathetic when we ourselves are in a situation. I have to muster my own internal fortitude and listen to my staff's complaints about the irritable, fearful patient and look at the person, see her loss of control, manage her expectations, and deal with her side effects no matter how trivial they are. I have to remember that at that time they are saying, "It really is all about me."

I cannot placate or diminish their concerns. It is one more way that these interactions are not normal conversations. These are not friends that you are trying to pat on the head. The patients are not relatives that you can just shrug off and say, "They are just emotional." This sacred time with them is meeting them at their most vulnerable moment, and it is a privilege to be here, really present and attentive to them and all of their concerns. Also remember that everything you say "can and will be held against you."

BARNEY

So **Barney** comes in for a work up and management of his lung cancer. He has very few teeth and is quite disheveled. He kind of reminds me of a Gabby Hayes character. He is a no-nonsense, get to the point kind of man.

He says, "This here's the deal, Doc. I feel like crap now. You're gonna make me feel worse, and I am gonna die anyway, so let's not waste each other's time. I got to go fishin'."

I've got nothing.

CHARLIE

The war veteran survived guns, missiles, and nightmares for two years. This head and neck cancer from smoking, however, will be tough. It will make him cry. He'll be emaciated (he refused a feeding tube) and will vomit every day because he so poorly tolerates the chemotherapy. **Charlie** has had a difficult life. When he was honorably discharged, he had nowhere to go and lived on the streets. He cleaned up enough to get a minimum wage job and ultimately have a lady friend. He is alone now, losing all of that and back on the streets. We are trying to get him resources, but it is not at all easy. The side effects are awful. The food he can get, he can't eat. He did not get any prescriptions filled because he can't pay the copay.

I say, "Charlie we have to get this nausea under control."

He says, "Doc, don't bother with the medications, I am going to smoke dope."

Somehow that he can get his hands on. He comes in the next week, and it has worked. He's much improved, and his appetite is gaining too. There is no question marijuana can be medicinal and a great help in hard-to-treat cases. I even have had elderly ladies use it when their grandkids get it for them. As a cancer specialist, I am glad we finally approved medicinal marijuana in Florida; no one wants granny in jail for smoking "the dope."

MR. CORBETT

The younger man in the exam room is tapping furiously on his phone. I enter the room and introduce myself to his mother, who extends her hand and an eye-roll to me. I prop myself on the rolling stool and wait until he is done— actually it takes a while. I don't have a sign that requests phones be "powered down" in the office, but it is a courtesy to be ready. I am not a prima donna, so I get that your time is as valuable as mine, but the tech age lends itself to significant rudeness, if not dangerous multitasking. The funny thing in this case is the young man expects me to get on with the interview and discuss cancer treatment all the while he is engaged on the phone.

I finally interrupt and say, "**Mr. Corbett**, please put the phone down so I can examine you and discuss your care."

He is surprised and a little annoyed. His actions say, "How long will this take? My real life is waiting on the phone."

After the exam I show him the films of the kidney mass that was found on an ultrasound of his gallbladder for pain. It is a "serendipitous finding," and in many ways he is fortunate since it is 3 cm and just the upper pole of his kidney will have to be removed. I make the necessary arrangements with the urologic cancer surgeon for the surgery, taking into account the patient's busy schedule and travel for business.

Before he leaves, I tell him that "cancer is inconvenient, but his time invested now will be worth it. Paying attention to this part of your life is important,"

I usually try to not lecture patients. It's their life after all, but you would be surprised how many times I hear, "I can't leave school;" "I don't have any more time for vacation;" "I need to care for someone;" "I have a trip planned;" "I have children to care for." It happens every day, and I respect that cancer is terribly inconvenient. It can often be a blessing when it stops us and makes us take note of life. It can focus us with laser precision about what is real. I love the phrase "pay attention; this is important" and use it often.

JIM

"Nobody gets out of here alive."

A true statement, but somehow I stand as a life protector, and hopefully the work I do can make the living longer or better. Okay, that's what I tell myself. Sometimes I wonder if it's worth it. The patient, **Jim**, is a good example of quality versus quantity. He survived war, the loss of his wife to cancer, and a debilitating neurologic disease, and now he has a head and neck cancer. I have described how toxic the therapy is. He received an oral drug to go along with radiation, and his lips are bleeding, his face has a blistering rash, his mouth is filled with fungus (thrush), his throat is so sore he cannot drink water or swallow his own secretions.

How often I tell people we will medicate you and bring you through the fire, but really he looks at me like, "Are you kidding me? I can't swallow the pain pills or even a liquid form. I don't want a feeding tube. Don't tell me it's going to get better in a few weeks. I am miserable now."

I know if I can just get him through, he really will do well. Years ago, patients went into cancer centers and lay in a bed for six weeks with IVs and nursing care. Now we expect to give the same and frequently more aggressive treatment and have the patient manage on their own.

Jim says "I quit. This is torture, and I am miserable."

I feel helpless to ameliorate his pain. I have tried everything. Without the feeding tube, he is in trouble. I have given him IV fluids as an outpatient. He is on his way to the hospital for help. He is only 30% through his prescribed treatment. It troubles me to see his distress because I know I am giving him state-of-the-art care. But he really cannot tolerate it anymore. I will give him a break which will decrease his chance of beating this disease, but some patients do not have the support, internal fortitude, or desire to fight, fight, fight anymore. Why should I push him? I wonder if I should let him quit. I have to remind myself that just because the patient says "I do" at the outset does not mean they really can do.

Heather

The father sits quietly by his lovely daughter, **Heather**, holding her hand. He is her greatest supporter and has been her whole life. When the diagnosis of metastatic breast cancer came at 38 years of age—in the bone, in the liver, in the lung—her husband of ten years bolted. She came to Florida to get care near her father, and he is ready to be her champion, confidant, cheerleader, rock. I am grateful to have him on our team. This petite girl with the bald head, big chandelier earrings, hip jeans, and T shirt is also doing all that she can to put forth a brave act for him. They both know she is dying, and the question today is can we radiate her bones and help the pain. Her father and I leave the room so she can change before my exam, and he puts a strong trembling hand on my arm.

"Doc, I'd do anything to change places with her. She does not deserve this. She's my baby."

We've all heard the saying that grief is harder when a child dies before the elderly. It's not the "natural" way. He can barely contain his grief, and they are both unnaturally stoic in the face of this monster. I recommend counseling. They need to work out all the anger and frustration and then gain acceptance if possible. They also need ultimate end of life plans to be addressed, and they cannot do this alone. I cannot provide all that they need, but I can see it clearly, and I am as heartbroken for him as for her.

They agree and are relieved to be referred, to have a safe place to bring their fears and tears. It is all I can offer. She dies two months later, and I pray that they were able to heal the pain if not the disease.

MR. JACKSON

"Oh, cut me a break," I say to the elderly patient as I move the pack of cigarettes in his shirt pocket away so I can listen to his heart.

He smiles through the dense nicotine stains on his mustache, beard, and teeth and says, "Doc, it's my only vice!"

I quip back, "I highly doubt that, **Mr. Jackson!**" to which he chuckles.

It's a well-known and recently re-confirmed fact that patients who smoke during therapy for lung cancer have worse outcomes (less disease control and die sooner). I have realistic goals—unlike the obese doctor who barks at the equally or even less obese patient to lose weight. I've never smoked, but I've seen the addiction and the aftermath my entire career.

So I ask Mr. Jackson how many packs per day (as with alcohol, with cigarettes we always assume double the amount they confess to).

He says, "Three! But I am down from four."

I wonder if he has time for anything else. I then ask how long he's been smoking, and this is a first for me.

"70 years!"

Mr. Jackson is 75.

"Now that is not possible that you started at five years old," I say as I contemplate getting the MRI of the brain.

"Oh, yes it is, Doc. My Daddy had a corner grocery store, and customers would get me to steal cigarettes (they were sold individually then). They'd light one for me, and we'd all go out back and smoke. Been doin' it my whole life now."

We all remember being shocked by the little Asian toddler seen on the viral video smoking. I thought this probably happens more than we know. We come up with a reasonable plan to manage his disease, and he lights up as soon as he gets to his truck, happy that he's made it this long.

MR. SULLIVAN

I am looking at the CT scan of a man with a very protuberant abdomen as he is being scanned. I see the pancreatic cancer, the belly filled with fluid (ascites), and the liver filled with tumor. At this time, I am still a resident and have gone out of town to help the practice of another doctor. I am doing the work of planning the radiation, which usually starts with a CAT scan through the area of disease so we can do the dosimetry of applying dose to the area for treatment. I have not met Mr. Sullivan myself. This was decided by the attending physician.

I ask the tech to stop the scan. I enter the room and look at the patient. I have the patient sit up on the table and introduce myself. I ask him what he likes to do, and he is surprised.

He says, "Doc, I love to fish. That's where I'd be if I was not here now."

I say, "**Mr. Sullivan**, I am going to write you the best prescription I have and that is to go fishing every day you can and do not come back here. You should not be spending any time in this department."

He knows what that means, and his eyes fill with tears as he softly says, "Thanks, Doc. I really appreciate that."

Sometimes giving the patient permission to live as they want is the best prescription we can fill. We often get so wrapped up in the frenzy of the process: diagnosis, planning, treatment; it is a challenge every day to remind myself to take those precious seconds and really look at the patient—helping them decide what they want and letting them know that it's okay to not want "everything done."

Miss Gladys

The elderly lady with the permed, teased, helmet hair sat very stiff and proper on the exam table. She looked over her bifocals, and I thought I was about to get a scolding. She never had healthcare because she never was "sick." This was foreign territory, unlike most of her friends who could lavishly describe every ache and pain and operation and symptom. She was stalwart.

I asked this lifelong librarian, as part of the history, when her symptoms started. She said that she found it difficult to sit on the tiny wooden stool at story time for the children. She has an anal cancer, truly "out the wazoo." She could not be more horrified. She is a virgin, and I have to examine her pelvis with the speculum. She will be poked and prodded and scanned and suffer every indignity which will further convince her that she was right to avoid medical care.

Miss Gladys requires chemo and radiation. She goes through treatment without a complaint—highly unusual since it can be very painful due to the reaction in that area. She wonders why this is all necessary since the pain is even worse during therapy. Ultimately she returns after many weeks. We examine her, and the tumor is gone.

She peers right at me over those same spectacles and severely says, "Don't ever do that to me again!"

MR. STILL

The patient is a dream. His wife is a sweetheart. Their daughter must have someone else's genes because she is a nightmare. Just the mention of her name and the entire staff trembles. I understand that she is "overseeing care" for her father since she is "in healthcare" and she wants power. But while we are managing **Mr. Still's** complex case, she is interfering. A cautionary tale. One doctor has already fired them. She is demanding and inappropriate. There are so many times as a doctor that you must exhibit the patience of a saint, but even I had just about had it. The daughter called and reamed my staff out over an appointment time that was inconvenient for her. The insults and tirades were completely inappropriate, but we were putting up with a lot for the sake of the ailing patient.

Finally, after one particularly brutal episode, I took the patient and his wife aside. I said, "Mr. Still, I must ask you to keep you daughter from my staff. She is bullying them (and him as well). I have a wonderful team, but if they are not living up to her expectations, then I suggest you all go elsewhere. They are my staff, not hers. I do not have to treat you. I can discharge you. But I will not have my staff abused by anyone."

I have had to stand up to inappropriate patients and families before, but this was the first time I was really firing a patient. We agreed that he and his wife would come in from now on without the daughter.

Even though there is great upheaval when a family member is ill, basic principles of kindness remain. Some people think that the squeaky wheel… But in fact, frequently these patients get less care and are discharged quickly.

I believe that advocates are important, but bullying is never appropriate. Sometimes I'll say, "Medication for everyone!" And I am not kidding.

Rachael

When I opened the exam room door, I was so surprised to see the lovely lady waiting. She was the wife of a former patient who had died 18 months before. She has been diagnosed with an early stage breast cancer, finally having time for her own healthcare. Many patients have gone through some significant life stressors, which can be contributing factors to their own diagnoses. Rachael was one of them. She had been with her husband every day through the radiation and chemo, and now she would have to come daily for her own treatments. She felt, however, that we had become part of her family, and she was very comfortable about the journey.

Midway through treatment she became very, very tired, and the fatigue was significant. I checked a chest x-ray and thyroid studies and put her on an antidepressant, but it continued.

So one day in the exam room, I sat down in front of her and said, "**Rachel**, I know that you are 50, but you have not gone through menopause. Is there any possible way you could be pregnant?"

Her eyes got enormous, and she finally nodded and said she'd had a "one night stand and did not even think to use any birth control because when her husband was alive he'd had a vasectomy."

We held the radiation and waited a long, agonizing 24 hrs for the blood test to return. She collapsed into my nurse's arms when the next day we told her it was negative. We were all thrilled, but it could have gone either way.

In her European accent, she sweetly said, "I am swearing off men completely!"

I said, "How about until the radiation is over?"

She said, "Okay, that makes more sense."

JOSEPH

At one time, I am sure the elderly man with the bright orange cap on his head was a master of industry. Now his granddaughter holds his hand and tries to recount the events over the past three weeks. At first he just had mild nausea. It was distracting when he was reading or playing bridge or doing crosswords. Eventually it was a constant companion. He told his son, and the snowballing events started to gain momentum.

He now has stitches in his scalp from the surgery to remove a glioblastoma grade-4 tumor. We are discussing radiation and chemo. The same questions arise: "How did this happen?" "Is it inherited?" "Were there signs earlier?" The reality is that if someone has not died of a heart attack by the age of 70, there is a 1-in-2 chance for men and a 1-in-3 for women that they will have cancer. Hence the average age of my patients is 73. Was this temporal lobe tumor from cell phone use, high intelligence, exposure to toxins? Someday these questions will have answers, but what does it matter now? The momentum is forward. He is eager to move on and get this business over with.

The interesting component of this discussion today is what's not said: the total defeat in his eyes, heightened by the perched hat. He cannot fathom that this is how it will end. Maybe we all hope to go quietly and quickly in the night. No fanfare, drama, or pain. This is a total insult to him and to his dignity. I ask the family to leave us alone, and there is a gasp of relief as they exit the room. I ask Joseph what he wants to do, and I am not surprised by the answer.

"Doc, I don't want to spend the time I have left coming in here every day even if you can extend my life. My brain is my power, and I greatly fear being a vegetable. What I need from you is to convince my family that I do not have to go through with this."

Once again I am faced with the tougher discussion of no treatment rather than just forging ahead. I tell Joseph to go home and make all the preparations with his will, banking, affairs, etc. I tell all my patients, "I don't know how long I am going to live. How can I possibly know how long you will? But I do know that we should all be prepared all the time."

Good advice; if it seems cowardly, so be it. It's the truth. So I tell Joseph it will probably be a few months 'til the end, but he can change his mind and come back anytime. For the family, I also advise them that it is his decision to hold treatment for now but that I am here anytime he wants to return.

Some of the inconsiderate ones pipe up: "But what will happen?" "How long will he have?" "Doesn't he have to get treated?" "Isn't this giving up?"

Joseph just rolls his eyes.

I say, "Your father knows exactly what he is choosing, and we need to respect his decisions." I am glad I do not have to go home in that car.

CONNIE

The recorder (without my permission) goes on, the notebook and pens come out, and we are on! This is a woman with a research background. If she can intellectualize and research enough, maybe she can make this go away. It won't be that simple. It is recurrent breast cancer, even after chemo and hormone treatment. When I review the history, something jumps out. Why did she have immediate reconstruction and never get radiation? The exact path to disease recurrence is not always so linear, but in this case, it is clear. She had multiple tumors in the breast, had a mastectomy and then reconstruction with an implant, and chemotherapy. She did not see a radiation oncologist, and with the implant in, the cosmetic results would be compromised after radiation.

Many patients want to get off the table like nothing happened. It does not work that way. The reconstructed tissue does not feel the same as a breast, or look the same. I am a cancer care specialist. I do not under any circumstances want to compromise the cancer operation in favor of cosmetics. Let's treat the cancer first.

For **Connie**, I can't say any of this. I tell her the tumors that are now growing over the implant need to be resected. The implant comes out and we do the radiation and change the hormone therapy she is getting. A good plan. In the one hour consultation, I spent 15 minutes on this direct approach. The discussion about redoing the implant and the cosmetics took the remaining 45 minutes. I have to allow that every patient comes with their own value system. She may have avoided this entirely with radiation the first time. Now I have insight into what her discussions had been five years ago and how she got to this point. She scribbles down my recommendations, states she will further research this, and get back to me.

I think the decision is fairly simple. Everything she reads will make this clear. But even if she replays this tape over and over, it is not the intelligent, thoughtful, research driven decision. It is emotional, and I have to give her time to process that. Sometimes doctors will want to tap, tap, tap the patient on the head and say, "Am I getting through? Is anyone up there listening?" But sensitivity is a crucial element of cancer treatment. We are always reminded that the patient, no matter how stubborn or resistant, or in denial, is the most important part of the team.

AGATHA

"You are not going to thank me for this," says the referring surgeon. "She is really tough and does not obey anything I say or take the treatment I have offered. Well, she's all yours now. Don't say I did not warn you!"

Wow! I think this will be more than interesting. I have not received a call like that in eons. So I am at least prepared as I enter her room.

She's a retired nurse who has a chest wall recurrence following a mastectomy, but this one is covering an entire half of her chest. It is a nasty, , massive disease that she now is willing to see if radiation will help. Again, you could have seen this coming. The original breast cancer was neglected, and when she had the mastectomy, she refused immediate chemotherapy and radiation to keep it under control. We are only six months later, and it is a mess. There is denial, and then there is delusion.

Agatha tells me what she is willing to accept and we come up with a plan, but still the chemo and hormones are refused. I have cajoled, begged, and brought her husband into the discussion, but we are going nowhere. After weeks of radiation, the tumor is worse. What had been covered by skin is now exploding. I am heartsick for her. It is painful and a nightmare. Now she wants to talk to a surgeon to see if the entire thing can come out—impossible. Frequently, patients do not know what they are asking for. When they bargain for less, they have to accept the consequences, and unfortunately they don't realize how awful they can be. Sometimes I am really dismayed by their reaction when they act like they had no idea. Really, people, listen to your docs.

Okay, let's have a discussion about what you are willing to go through, but some of that is the downside of not doing anything. We are not going to all go "gently into that good night." Sometimes it is going to be a nightmare that perhaps, just perhaps, we could have avoided.

Dorothy

Dorothy was treated for bone lesions from breast cancer. It was a simple treatment with radiation and a bone-strengthening IV drug once each month as well as a change in hormone therapy. So I am surprised to see her in my waiting room weeks after therapy is over. Her husband is reading the paper, having coffee, and watching the news on our TV.

I pull up a chair and ask Dorothy how she is doing.

She says, "Great, all the pain is gone."

So I venture further while she fits the puzzle pieces together with satisfaction. "Is there something I can do for you?" My staff tells me she is coming here every day. Did she miss the point of being discharged from my care?

Dorothy looks up and smiles. She says, "Doc, when I was coming here, it was a happy time for me. You would think most people would be happy to get out of here, but this is my social life now. I sit at this puzzle table, and other patients come by and sit, and we talk. I give them encouragement and listen to their woes. I love doing the puzzles, and it's an outing for my husband and me. If you don't mind, I'd like to come here for a while."

I told Dorothy she and her husband were welcome anytime and that I was sure the other patients looked forward to seeing her as well. Patients do develop an attachment. One even came by several times to "visit the machine." She said that after spending 35 days with it, she missed seeing the tomotherapy unit. That was a first for me. My staff is wonderful in letting the patients know we consider them part of our family. For those that feel a need to be engaged, we give them information on volunteering and support groups which can be a very helpful way for people to share this life altering experience. It's a good thing patients like to donate puzzles so we can have a new one every day!

MR. BUCHMAN

"I can't go out there!" This is our medical assistant. "He's always hugging me, yew! What's up with that?"

There is something called transference, and patients will occasionally view us as a family member. Many patients see me as their daughter, sister, or mother, and it's natural when people are trying to put some controls around you, not just to view you as their doctor. We are very warm and supportive here, so hugs are free! Unfortunately, some people take advantage of the nurturing and feel that their life-threatening situation should allow for certain liberties.

That's the problem at hand with **Mr. Buchman**. He is rather unkempt and wearing a stained T-shirt and mud-covered boots. I have had to tell patients to bathe or remove their filthy shoes outside the treatment room before getting on the table or provide them with a cloth and towel and escort to the rest room. Not everyone has the same sense of decorum, and so we have to "help them" get along with us. My concern today however, is Mr. Buchman's behavior!

This patient, is just plain inappropriate. The nurse tells me that she is intentionally avoiding him since he seeks her out and gives her a hug almost every day. Her demeanor is very sweet and she does not want to offend anyone, but it's going to take intervention. I have seen patients ask my nurses for a date, call them after hours, give them notes, come by to visit and hug them too much. This is not a singles bar. This is a professional healthcare business, and it is not okay. I have told patients that I will discharge them if they do not behave. I have admonished patients to stop flirting, telling them that the staff is here to care for them and not for their amusement. Just like patients or families that are overbearing or rude, there are other ways I have responsibility to protect the staff.

Once a patient was teasing about a procedure that the female technologist had to perform while treating his cancer, and she told me his conversation made her uncomfortable. I put the hammer down fast and the next time he came in, and for the remainder of the therapy, I sent our 6'2", Chinese, male physicist in the room to perform the procedure.

MRS. HERNANDEZ

Mrs. Hernandez is a small, squat, blond, vivacious firecracker and 82 years old. She is from Puerto Rico and does not speak English. Her daughter is translating, and I could see the large, dark owl-like eyes just terrified about the treatment for breast cancer. She will do well, but having had minimal healthcare, this is a very threatening experience for her. The doctor who is introducing her to me includes that Mrs. H. is a cousin of a famous young singer/dancer, and I see the patient's face light up.

I take her hand and lift her from the chair. I say, "I don't believe you are related to that performer. Let me see you dance!"

She starts gyrating her hips and giggling and twirling around. The serious conversation is over. I describe to her daughter what has to be done and the boring, dry details of it all. Each week as the patient is seen during treatment, as soon as I walk in the room, she gets up and dances for us. When she finishes her therapy, she tells us that she'll miss coming because every day was like a party and she'll miss the attention. She's related to S….. And a performer in her own right!

I told the daughter and patient that patients come to us for all sorts of reasons. Frequently it's not just to treat the disease. Those patients that are "well" and not debilitated give us all the uplift and energy we need to manage the rest of our day and difficult cases. This is the case with Mrs. Hernandez; we needed her here more than she needed us.

ELSIE

Elsie looks like my 4th grade teacher. She is round, grey, and very sweet. What is a surprise is that, at 65 years of age, she maintains a strong, guarded, protectionist view of her large breasts. She had breast cancer years ago and now has a recurrence. When she had her first mastectomy, she had immediate reconstruction. Therefore she has never been without some "breast tissue." Elsie is adamantly opposed to having the implant removed and having any further surgery for skin recurrence. Breast cancer is sneaky and can come back years later. It is unfair if you've had a breast removed that it can still return. After all, isn't that the trade off? In Elsie's case, because of the implant, she refused to have radiation when she was first diagnosed, which may have avoided this recurrence.

We've seen this before. Radiation can change the configuration of the capsule of any implant, making it very unacceptable cosmetically. Therefore I prefer to radiate the chest wall if the patient's disease requires it (which her's did) and then have the implant placed about six months later.

She has now had the implant removed and is sitting with big wads of cloth tucked into her bra. She has not had a fitting for prosthesis. It will be very heavy since it will match her opposite breast, which is very large. She is grieving the loss of the implant but attempting to come to grips with the change in her anatomy.

Today she says, "I have decided to not have another reconstruction. God is telling me something about my vanity. My husband and I decided that it is more valuable to walk on the beach and eat an apple and spend time together than suffer through another surgery just to put balloons in my chest."

She is saying these words but may not own them.

So I say, "Let's do the cancer treatment first, and then in 6 months if you want to reconsider the implant, we'll discuss it again."

I am all about not closing the door on options for patients. When they know that they can change their mind, that decisions are not set in stone, that life is long and requires reassessment ongoing, they are more likely to be relieved. There's a lot of pressure in cancer care, and so many times the stress is not the cancer.

POLLY

Chemo-brain! It is a real phenomenon. It's reported more often by women than men. But it's a non-discriminatory side effect to chemotherapy. **Polly** is an African American woman who has worked hard to advance her career and be a role model for her son. The single mother is now in upper management for a company and working on her master's degree.

Here is the problem: When Polly started her radiation, she had completed the necessary chemotherapy for node positive breast cancer and had a mastectomy and now is undergoing the final course of her treatment. She states today that her forgetfulness and hesitation has become dramatically worse. Even simple issues are difficult to resolve, and her memory for very recent recall is severely hampered. She had to actually request a demotion. She admitted to her COO that she could not do the job but wanted to stay with the company. She was completely demoralized. She was feeling like a failure, and all the treatment and stress contributed to her downfall.

This is the first time anyone has addressed "chemo brain" with her. The mental cloudiness, the disconnect between thought and words, and the lack of attention span or comprehension are all part of the syndrome's reality. We also find it in men with prostate cancer on hormones and women who are on long-term hormonal manipulation for breast cancer.

I applaud Polly's resolve to stay with the company since, if she can regain function, she'll have a real possibility of getting her job back. I am also encouraged that she is flexible enough to modify her life according to need and ability. That practice will serve her longer than just a management position.

GERTRUDE

"I just thought as you grow older, your thighs get bigger!"

Okay, that may actually be true for women, but in **Gertrude's** case, the only part growing was a grapefruit-sized tumor under her buttock. It was large, hard, and non-tender. It was actually her gynecologist who found it when she was placed "in position" for her pap test.

She chuckled, "It almost hit him in the head, flapping around like that!"

Good thing she has a sense of humor. She'll need it as she undergoes radiation then surgery for an aggressive and rare muscle tumor. These tumors can occur in the arms and legs (extremities) or be hidden from view deep behind the kidneys (retroperitoneal). They are usually treated by radiation and surgery, sometimes requiring amputation of a limb! There is no known common cause. Angiosarcomas can be caused by radiation; sometimes scar tissue can mutate and form sarcomas. Fibromas and desmoid tumors can become large masses before they are finally evaluated by an MRI. For the most part, they just pop up like a lump under the skin.

In another case, a young, male construction worker was told he had a lipoma (a common, benign, fatty growth) until it became harder and larger and a sarcoma was found on biopsy.

As I told Gertrude, not every lump or bump is cancer, but in this case, thank goodness for the gynecologist. She states that she cannot wait to see if her thighs get thinner with the treatment. If that's what gets her through!

CHRISTINE

"Just let me start by saying I was an oncology nurse and I like to direct my care. I want IV fluids a few times a week from this company, blood work drawn weekly to include tumor markers, my treatments at a time each day convenient to me, and I never expect to wait more than a few minutes for you!"

Whew! I don't even know her diagnosis, but I know her management. This patient must control whatever she can if we are to have success. I have to prescribe and administer, but this patient needs and should be given the opportunity to manage some aspects of this plan. I have no problem with that. I am not a doc who is a dictator—my way or the highway. I understand that every patient manages their issues as individuals, and I may change the disease response but not the personality. For as many patients as intellectualize the disease—read everything they can on the internet, converse with friends, see several specialists, others say, "Hey, Doc, whatever. You're the doc, and you know best."

Therefore I am forever changing with the dynamic in front of me. For **Christine**, controlling what she could when she has a deadly disease and feels out of control is her right. Getting the staff to go along with a headstrong patient, however, is another thing.

In an unusually irritable moment, one tech said maybe we should give her the keys so she can treat herself! When you watch the dynamic with their families, like a husband rolling his eyes or a meek, nervous daughter, you want to help the entire process as much as possible. If I take her control, I may take her spirit. So instead I gently bargain for what I need to get it all done, to treat her disease but let her feel that it was all her doing. Much like any relationship, the doctor-patient one can be tenuous and requires mutual respect. As long as there is understanding and give and take on both sides, I work with every personality. I believe I have a high EQ (emotional quotient). I get that from my parents and from being the middle child, a lucky combination for success in these interactions. Finally, after several weeks, Christine did well, remained in control, and we all got the job done without the tech tossing her the keys.

JENNY

"Doc, my back hurts!"

"But we're treating your mouth," I say.

"I know, but my back is killing me."

I work with the techs to see if it's the position, not enough padding, the bumpers, the table, etc., etc., etc. Finally, since we can't seem to get it right, I ask, "Did this start with our treatment?"

Jenny says, "Oh, no, I've had this problem for 30 years!"

Now this is not the first time, so why am I always blindsided by this? Patients frequently see their docs for one reason but expect that visit to be magical and resolve every other issue. It's like getting a pap test and then having a heart attack a week later.

The patient says, "I was just at the doctor. How did this happen?"

My advice: When you go to the doctor, remember they are human and not mind readers. Make a list of what is bothering you then address them one by one at the visit. If nothing can be done, perhaps accept it as part of living (I dislike saying aging). With Jenny, her back pain was short-lived. When her mouth pain started from the side effects to treatment, the pain medicine I gave her took care of both. That was easy!

LILA

"I gonna live until I die and no longer!"

Funny that a nurse-patient said that to me 20 years ago. How very profound now from this tiny 92-year-old, white–haired, toothless, sweet-grinning great-great-grandmother.

I looked into her clouded eyes and said, "I got nothing!"

Really, what do you say? Okay, I can give her treatment for this small tumor and probably make her miserable in the process. She is tired and does not want to get dressed to leave the house every day (as evidenced by her housecoat, slippers, and uncombed hair). Her caretaker is with her. The rest of the family moved away, are working, or are already deceased.

The caretaker shrugs her shoulders and says, "I was told to bring her."

Lila is not going to die from the tumor, so I don't see any reason to get hospice involved. What I need to do is convince the referring physician that she is just fine for her remaining time and that I am always here to help if things go south. That's a good plan: leave the door open but respect their wishes. I say goodbye and that I am sorry that we won't get to be entertained by her wit and wisdom each day. There's a lot going on in there, and she should share her humor.

HAZEL

"How is it possible that my wife has cancer? I never even heard the word until I was 30. Come to think about it, I had not heard heart disease until then either."

Now I am just wondering where the rock he was hidden under is. I explain that it is common to get blindsided. As we get older, our life changes and we become the next generation. I saw Michael Douglas on Oprah talking about how his life changed after the diagnosis of cancer. It's really an awakening to a new life. I tell **Hazel** and her husband what I have learned: At first life is about education, having a family, providing, making a home. Then we get complacent with our own lives and frequently grieve the loss of children to making their own livelihood sometimes far away. Suddenly we are the next generation, and the issues are very different. People behave differently. One of my coworkers says at 50 she became invisible.

We start to see some friends and relatives have health problems. First it's the knees, then maybe a "mini stroke" maybe a small breast or colon cancer. Then everything starts to escalate in a big way. A friend or peer dies, has a by-pass, gets an overwhelming cancer and the next time you see them they are bald. People move to be with their children, not to help out and babysit or be there for a birth, but because they need help to navigate their healthcare.

When they look at nursing homes for their parents, they evaluate with a more critical eye as if to say, "Would I like it here?" If you are reading this and becoming a senior (or super senior!) admit that you are doing this. Hold those car keys tighter—actually I am thinking about making a second pair and hiding them. Hope I remember where I put them.

STEPHANIE

The patient is lovely, pulled together, and professionally dressed with her appointment book and gold pen in hand. She is writing down everything I say about the treatment for breast cancer while her husband fires off questions nonstop. He is in the medical field and has researched the heck out of this—hyper-intellectualizing this disease. After all, this is their first time dealing with a major life crisis. They have had a gilded life to date and are ready for a jet-setting retirement. They are a lovely, beautiful couple. She is in control. He is traumatized. I want to say that no matter what he questions or I answer I cannot make this go away. It happens so often. Just like the child that falls down the steps—the pediatrician will say, "The child is fine—give the mother a sedative!"

I have to manage information for the spouse who is in denial. There are no comforting words. He won't hear them. He wants this problem over and now. **Stephanie** is cringing. She is the one to actually go through this, but as with so many patients, they try to protect their loved ones. At times like this, the only answers are to give all the answers. If you shortcut something, they come back to it like he did. If you "blow something off," they want to investigate that more. There is absolutely no placating. Unfortunately, this can interfere with getting the patient's needs met.

In today's case, her needs are really to protect her husband, and so I give into that. I will try to find a time during another visit to listen to her, help her, answer her, comfort and advise her. Today it really is about him. I get that quickly and so they have a fruitful visit. She winks at me as they leave. I admire her courage and strength, enough for both of them.

HARVEY

Harvey is a tall, skinny, African American man in his 80s. He is here because his family doctor thought radiation would help the pain in his shoulder from metastatic prostate cancer. He has worked on a farm here in the South his whole life and has no education and a poor understanding of his disease. It is very confusing how a problem in his prostate is affecting his shoulder. I lay out the information and explanations then tell him how we can help him if he comes in several days, 15 minutes per day, to get radiation. The toothless, wide-eyed look he gives me is priceless. I have to laugh out loud because something I do every day sounds so unusual and almost crazy to him. That's probably true for most doctors' visits.

Of course, if it's something like, "Doc, this hurts," and the doc says, "Okay, I'll cut it out," then that seems reasonable. Something as complicated as using radiation to change the DNA of the cells to allow cancer to die off and help the pain etc., etc., etc. must be a very foreign idea. And occasionally, even I have to admit it seems farfetched.

Harvey just gets up, shakes my hand, smiles, and says, "Nope!" Guess he told me.

SAM

I am often asked, "How do you do this?"

People don't mean the radiation; they mean treating people with cancer all day, every day. I ignore the emotional toll, but occasionally that stinking, defeated gremlin creeps in. Today is one of those times. I just received a notice that one of my patients died. Although this is expected since many patients I see have extensive diseases, I am always moved. I think of the parents, spouses, children left behind. I am inspired by the courage, their personal stories, the drama, their internal fortitude, and occasionally just their ability to get up in the morning.

Today I learned that a young man died who touched all our hearts. **Sam** came to me with an extensive cancer. He had surgery and then received radiation and chemotherapy. I first met him a year ago. He lived longer than expected because, even with significant disease, young people do not have other co-morbidities. They have strong hearts, lungs, and kidneys. They usually die from the cancer and not "side effects" like pneumonia, blood clots, or heart failure. They "hang on," still expecting against the odds to at least get to see middle age. I have chosen to limit my patients to adults over 18. I cannot bear the management of children. But as a mother and grandmother, I am deeply moved by these "adult children."

Sam was 34. For unknown reasons, he developed a cancer. Sam had low-set ears, a wide glabellum between the eyebrows, unusual body habitus, and unfortunately, mental retardation. Sam worked every day and was well liked and cheerful. He did not have Down's syndrome, and in today's world the chromosomal abnormality could have been mapped. Sam was just living his life when he had severe abdominal pain and the sky fell on his poor mother. She was 65 and appeared to be in good health, but single parents of challenged children worry about a future for their child without them. Now her personal issue is heartache.

The last I'd heard from Sam was two months ago. We called him to come in for his appointment. He said he had to work, and since he was cancer "free," he did not need to be seen. One of his other physicians had him undergo testing and there had been no sign of disease on the x-rays. In a way, I was glad for Sam that he lived his last weeks "well." Whatever aspect of the cancer he succumbed to is irrelevant. It was more about living normally. A lesson for us all is his sweet innocence.

SHARON

"These women all need a makeover!" The 30-something gorgeous model, **Sharon**, is coming from the waiting room and into our office for a very deadly disease. The life expectancy is short, but she is focused on anything but herself. We do get through the treatment and recognize that part of her healing is a need to connect and to do something for others. So we set up a makeover clinic for any of our patients who wish to participate. She teaches them about makeup and how to strut a bald head or find the right wig. She shows them what to do about the clothes that are hanging instead of fitting, how to be empowered and not look like victims. She is sweet, tough, and great fun, a ball of self-assured, beautiful energy.

At first the other patients do not realize she has cancer. When she whips off her wig and shocks them, they open their hearts to her. Sharon has taken on this project with great vigor, and everyone whom she touches has adopted her. Sharon has no father and an estranged mother. She has a boyfriend but no siblings or children. She is really alone. Sharon has found a way to make her own "family." Whenever these women come in for visits, they ask about her. They have gone to lunch, connected on Face book, and chatted. It has been a whirlwind. It is a super lesson for us all. Create your own "family." Not everyone is blessed with the full support team. This was her personal way to find them, and she did it in one night. She is not manipulating them, she just saw a need and filled it, and now this group boosts their feel good hormone, oxytocin, by connecting regularly. I am thrilled about this. She is doing better than expected. Finding something and some people to live for definitely boosts the immune system. I am so very proud of Sharon, and I want her to be at that end of the Gaussian curve where some people live against the odds. (Note: Thee years later, she is still amazing!)

AMELIA

Amelia is terrified. She is here with her loving, doting, devoted husband of 35 years. They have both battled cancer. She has metastatic disease, and I treated her at first two years ago. She did well and has maintained "control" for that time. When it is time to scan, she loses her own self-control.

The nurse looks at me and says, "Her heart rate is 120!"

I say that it is psychologically induced. We are going to "look the devil in the eye" again and see how much the disease has grown. Lucky for her today, there is minimal change. We have options for her, and I offer them but try to interject that with this disease, maybe "less is more." The challenge in treating this disease is its complexity and then the added variable of each and every individual—their physical, psychological, and emotional makeup. Try to decide: Should we micromanage? Can she tolerate a wait and see approach? I thought in the six months between our visits that she had gotten on with her life. She tells me she has a terrible life, but she is perfectly "normal"—no pain, no symptoms, nothing.

I am learning another lesson today. Amelia needs to be under treatment to be happy. She does not want to live her life and enjoy every moment with this disease hanging over her head. She has been incapable of treasuring each day. After an hour of discussion, the light bulb finally goes on for me and I agree to treat her. She is visibly relieved. Her heart rate comes down. She is empowered. Even though I thought I improved her life by a watch and see attitude (after two years of intense therapies), she was unable to live that life well.

Therefore she will start retreatment in a few weeks even though I know I am not extending her days. This may well be a waste of time, but since there is a very slight chance it will help, she is a willing participant. There are no secrets here. I lay it out for her and her husband. They both are relieved, and I learn the lesson to listen and avoid interjecting my own value system.

GREGORY

"Hey, Doc, come here. I need to tell you something." I lean over closer to the elderly man's face because I think he wants to whisper (in front of his family). Instead he shouts like I am the one hard of hearing: "Don't waste my time! I am 88 years old, and I ain't got that much of it left!"

I have already switched gears from Amelia who wants me to "waste her time," to this. Since I am so close, I peer at his forehead. I say "I don't see an expiration date up there, so settle down and let's come up with a plan."

He chirps, "Okay!"

He knows I got the point, and I promise to not waste his time. **Gregory** enjoys every day of treatment, all the attention he gets from the staff and interaction with other patients. He has stories to share and acts like he is coming for a social. It's the highlight of his year, and he looks brighter and more alive than when I first met him. Guess we are not wasting his time!

STACEY

Stacy is holding a "basketball" under her gown. It is tucked under her left arm, and she carries it against her chest with her right hand.

She is in her 50s and starts her story with, "15 years ago, I felt a lump. I never wanted to do anything about it until it caused a lot of pain last month. Now I need help."

I gingerly move the gown aside and I am met with the largest tumor in the breast I have ever seem. Breast cancers neglected can be messy. This one filled the breast and pumped it up like a big ball, hard and tender. She could not lie down with it; her clothes could not fit well over it, so she wore a man's T shirt. The pain was evident.

It's tragic when patients who could have been easily managed choose this route of non-care. Now we have to pull out all the guns. She'll need heavy chemo, scans, surgery, and then radiation. She worked in the healthcare field, and I've seen this before. Sometimes these individuals', knowing what is ahead, are the hardest to convince that treatment now rather than later is the best.

I do not admonish her; I do not look surprised. I quietly take her hand and say, "Stacy, here is your problem. As much tumor as you have, it is still not enough to kill you. If I thought you would die soon from this, we would manage your pain and that would be that. But this tumor is just in an appendage. It has not traveled to your organs (dire sights), so you won't die of lung or liver failure, heart failure or brain mets. This will be a long, unnecessary purgatory. The flames will lick you and never go out. It will be very slow. You are young, so you have a good heart and those patients take the longest to die from their disease. So my best recommendation, understanding how you feel, is to advise you to receive at least a first dose of chemo. Then at last you will know what you are doing and not run from treatment due to fear. Perhaps you will be pleasantly surprised and accept treatment. Go with the first dose; you can always stop."

She left in tears, grateful for the understanding. She made the appointments, and now I hope she keeps them.

KEBBY

"I am fat and I don't have any eyebrows!" The 37-year-old patient, **Kebby,** has completed chemo and radiation and is in for follow-up. The breast cancer issue is controlled, but now she is living with the side effects of treatment. We spend her visit discussing what beauty-enhancing products may help and how to start exercising. She leaves happy with her cosmetic shopping list, and I am happy that as a female I can help her. She is to start a walking exercise program. Once a patient finishes treatment, they need something to focus on. They need to find new goals. Treating cancer, showing up for therapy, kept them on a path that has suddenly disappeared. It's good to give them direction, support, and concrete goals for living between visits.

PATRICIA

Patricia has finally grown her hair back after chemotherapy. I am sorry to have to tell her it will all disappear for several months once again. She has a type of lung cancer (Small or Oat Cell) that spreads rapidly throughout the body. This is the cancer from which people used to die within six week of diagnosis. With the advent of chemotherapy improvements, this disease is survivable even when stage IV.

Patricia only had the disease in her lung (limited disease) and therefore received chemo and radiation together. She did very well, and now it is time for another discussion. She is a candidate for "prophylactic" radiation to the brain. It is the only time radiation is given when there is no disease! Because the cells are small and spread rapidly, they can get into the brain, but due to a "blood brain barrier" that keeps chemo out, the brain becomes a "sanctuary site" for these cells. Up to 80% of patients with small cell lung cancer will develop brain mets unless we prophylactically radiate the brain.

Patricia went on a long train trip across the U.S. before we started this part of the process.

She said, "Doc, I was so thrilled to see the Grand Canyon, to go to the Hollywood Walk of Fame, to see Rodeo Drive. I realize that the world is so much bigger than my little cancer environment. Do whatever you must because when this is finally over, I will get out and live the life I never did before. I may not have much time, but I am done wasting it and over wallowing in self pity."

HERBERT

"Doc, whatever you do, don't let my husband know I called."

Once a patient has signed consent that we may share information or speak with a family member, it is perfectly legitimate to accept these calls, and sometimes they can be very helpful. After all, it is the spouse, significant other, daughter, etc. who are with these patients 24/7. They know what is going on and need to download, ask questions, express concern, or find out how long until the inheritance comes in! Today the call is from a loving wife at her wits end. Her husband, **Herbert**, has been battling lung cancer for eight years, so unusual for a disease whose two-year life expectancy is 20%, and now finally the end is near. How unfortunate that the efforts they have both expended—the expectations for a good life not met, the drama of loss of work, the lack of play, and the loss of house and health—has taken such a toll. They, like others, thought the good life comes at retirement. He was five years from that time. He won't see that. He finally left even the menial job he was now doing because he could not get out of bed. He is still on chemotherapy, but it's not working any more.

Now her loving husband, to whom she is so totally devoted, is dying, but before he does, he has become aggressive. He is not just angry, he is mean. How often I hear this from family and spouses. It's not always the disease; it may be pain, brain dysfunction, medications. So I advise her to bring him in today. When they arrive, she sheepishly tells me that she let him know about the call. The insight the family gives me is so helpful. How would I know when he is so sweet with the staff and me that he is screaming at her at night? I am so saddened by these turns of events, seeing them as I do in patients who need that person now more than ever and knowing they cannot help themselves.

This is where the anti-anxiety medications, the morphine, and the anti-depressants come in. I frequently advise counseling for the surviving person. I want everyone to know this is normal. It does not reflect your care or the patient's "evilness." It is part of illness and too often part of dying. I advise Herbert in front of his wife that the end is near, that any treatment other than managing pain should be stopped. What difference does it make if they are miserable for a few more weeks or comforted for a few days? It's a lot of difference to the survivor. I want the patient to consider being less selfish, to stop holding on at all costs because it is killing both of them.

How to get this across delicately? I usually softly say, "I think it's time to consider comfort care. Let's see what we can do to help you feel more like yourself." Everyone usually understands that message. Some need me to say, "Please put your affairs in order, time is limited." I will often say, if pushed, "You have months (or weeks), not years."

The patient looks almost relieved today; his wife definitely is.

Dawna

"Please help me," her tiny voice and big eyes come from a large, over-300 lb. body.

Dawna has breast cancer growing in her bones. She has had this for a few years, and now all the inactivity has taken a toll, leaving her weak, in a wheelchair, obese from the chemo and steroids. Her hips and pelvis cannot tolerate any weight. Her family cannot lift her. She cannot go to the bathroom without a team. She is in pain whether in the bed or wheelchair. Nothing is comfortable, and the slightest movement sends a driving shock of pain visible on her face before she even cries out.

We gather around and try to get her positioned on the table for radiation, but the pain is too great. We try new pain meds and give her a few days, but she comes in no better, even as the narcotics increase and she becomes more somnolent. Finally, she is completely sedated and I think we will have success, but the terrible pain coursing through her wakes her up just as she is placed in position. I am at a loss. No radiation is going to get this managed.

Her plight is a continuous reminder of the ugliness of this disease. I am sick of it for her. Her family is beside themselves. They are dealing with this 24/7 and feeling helpless. We send her to the hospital for pain management. There she will be sedated, probably discharged to hospice. The admission is a sign that the end is near. Nothing more can help. Everyone should have the ability to be pain free, but this will require complete sedation. As much as the family wishes otherwise, there is relief. They just cannot take the burden any longer.

CHARLOTTE

"Go on vacation," I tell the young patient, her family, and husband.

I am all about trying to allow the patient to have a life. It's hard when you're in the midst of therapy and that becomes your life, to remember that the rest of the family is still trying to live! It sounds so obvious, but it is the one aspect of caring for patients that can get away from us. This is not a third-world country. Many other physicians are strict and want to keep the patients close to home—not me. If they have a problem while on vacation, they can go to the nearest ER and get care!

So now I have to confess it did not work out so well in this case. The call came in Saturday night. "Doc, she trashed the hotel room and cussed out her family and the staff," and all around created quite a chaotic time. The entire family is so upset and terrified. The young, professional woman has brain metastasis from lung cancer. **Charlotte** was placed on steroids and now has an acute steroid psychosis.

The agitation and aggressive behavior, out of character for these patients, shocks their loved ones, but there is almost nothing other than sedation that works until they recover. Finally, a week later, there is improvement. She is becoming more aware, less upset, and paranoid but is still not herself. Her husband hasn't slept all week. A few times she called the police, unknown to him until they showed up at the door.

You think how unfair all this is. At a time when there is so little time, it is such an insult to the injury. Enough is enough. The discussion you had just last week about how much more time there may be becomes a moot point.

The disease and its treatments are thieves, stealing the few good moments left. There is a sad realization from the family that there is no getting back to baseline. This happens so often: the patient on the ventilator, the stroke, the coma, the confusion, and so many manifestations of end stage. Just as you thought you could handle that the end is in the near future, the intervening time is lost too. There is a tornado effect of the disease now capturing the loved ones and friends and hurling them outward instead of toward the person who needs them most. It is a courageous family, husband, daughter who stands by and recognizes that the abuse, the words, the anger is not directed toward them but to this thing called cancer.

I just hope they can hold on for the rough ride. Her husband is trying his own remedy. He has pulled out the notes, cards, letters she has received over the past year and quietly sits with her, reading them, hoping he is making his way through to her normal self and giving her hope. So much sweet selflessness captures our hearts.

MR. COLLINS

It's the first time I am seeing this in my career. The very sweet middle-aged man is accompanied by his doting wife. He is in a wheelchair. I am asked to evaluate him for radiation to the brain. A few years ago, he had a kidney removed with "renal cell carcinoma." This disease now has several chemo agents used to help control it that have some degree of success, and he has been on some of them. He now has a tumor in the ventricle of the brain (choroid plexus) where renal cell cancers can "hide." That is not the interesting part.

I start to examine him, and he tells me he is blind in his left eye. I had not seen any tumors in the occipital lobe or even within the brain, but this seems to have come on recently. He went to an ophthalmologist who injected him for diabetic retinopathy. He states that he is now going blind in the right eye. I look at the scan again, and he actually has tumors behind the "globe" of the eye. Both eyes are involved, and this is causing the blindness.

That is the issue with metastatic disease. "Meta" means elsewhere. The cancer starts in one organ and then finds its way through the bloodstream or lymphatics to another. After I research this, I find that these orbital tumors, which we see in breast cancer and lymphoma, can be common in metastatic renal cell cancer. They are very sneaky and very devastating because there is no disease elsewhere. Now this cancer that started in a kidney is stealing his vision.

I ask his wife how they are managing. She took family leave to care for him. He is a big man, and to keep him from falling, he spends most of his time in a wheelchair so she can help him get around. He says it's a new life, this blindness, and the challenges are significant.

I saw him in the hallway a few days later and said, "Hello, **Mr. Collins**, do you remember me?" Then I added, "It's Dr. Dragun!"

I thought, "How would he know who this voice is?"

So now the staff talks to him by first stating their names since he cannot see them. (Funny that we also speak louder, although there is nothing wrong with his hearing).

One day, he said, "Hey, Doc, where's that cute young nurse of yours?"

I realize this is inappropriate but go along with him and chuckle that she's on vacation visiting family. The "cute young nurse" indeed has a sweet, lilting voice, which she uses to practice singing lullabies to her grandchildren. I won't destroy his fantasy.

MICHELLE

The patient has a drug and alcohol problem. It predated her diagnosis, so it's not prescription drugs, but she'd like nothing better than for all of the docs involved to be her providers. The dilemma here is the confusion they cause. She is in a battle royal with every member of the staff. We don't always get to choose our patients, and so the staff practices tolerance, understanding, patience, and fortitude and does a lot of acting.

Reasoning with a dependent person is near impossible. **Michelle** blames everyone for everything. "I got lost because that girl gave me the wrong directions. I did not get a call (she got three of them) about my appointment. I don't like this or that. I did not like that doc."

I know it's only a matter of time (probably when I refuse to give a prescription) before I'll be defiled too. We want her to be treated for the cancer. She needs this care. We try to refer for therapy, but she denies any problems. She states she is in recovery, but we all know that is false. I worry about how she gets here, so we provide transportation to keep her off the roads.

I think about the myriad people we see: all of them at some critical point in their lives. All struggling with past and present demons. They are carving out these 30 minutes per day to come into our "therapeutic" world. Sometimes it is sobering to realize what little impact we truly have. We cannot cure everything that is wrong. We cannot patch the family, fix the pain, wipe the tear, repair the marriage, raise the children, heal the heart, feed the hungry, exorcise the fears, or limit the drama. We are a tiny, narrow-as-a-thread slice on their pie charts.

Many of them exclaim our virtues; families return after a death and thank us for the care. Many positive reactions almost daily help us keep our chins up, and I have to thank these souls for giving us the encouragement we need. I am always grateful, remembering that my staff is mostly women who have chosen a difficult field. I could not do it without them.

DEBRA

The young woman on the table is absolutely terrified. She is only in her early 30s. She is trembling, crying, and can hardly speak. Her significant other brought her in to be evaluated for a mass in her neck which came on suddenly. I had sent her for a scan and a biopsy. It is Nodular Sclerosing Hodgkin's Disease. I review the scan in detail and advise her that chemotherapy will be first then radiation to follow, that she is "fixable" and her disease is controllable, and that she will start to feel better once she is treated.

She cannot hear anything. I think her teeth are chattering. She is lucky to have great support, or we would never have been able to get through this session. I am trying to lessen the blow, speak softly, and exude confidence. We have to carry her gently through this process. She was so scared that she stayed in bed all week and did not go to work, not a good thing. I like patients to work as long as their blood counts are good because it keeps life somewhat normal and keeps them from being a victim. It also helps pay their bills and maintain insurance so they can get the care.

We are going to get her on medication to help the depression and anxiety quickly. Fear is paralyzing. **Debra** feels it's all happening so fast. Sometimes the disease is ahead, and as we scramble to catch up, we leave the patient behind. Occasionally, given all the time in the world, the patient can't process what is happening. I prefer to just pick her up, throw her over our collective shoulders, and carry her through this to the other side. I have to remember this is about Debra, and if I do not give it time to sink in, we may treat the disease and destroy the patient. In this case, it will be better to get her on medication, take a few weeks, and then forge ahead. Baby steps are still steps.

GORDON

"When is this radiation out of my body?"

The man is in his 50s and had prostate treatment a year ago. Now I understand that there are long-term effects of treatment—sexual dysfunction, bowel and bladder problems—but he had none of those. He is just "wiped out." When we investigate, I am only left with the issue that he must have some degree of depression that has gone untreated. This happens often in patients undergoing therapy and then suddenly they are done and left to their own devices.

Other than medication, I prescribe exercise—a great choice to heal mind, body, and spirit. As we talked about this, it became clear that **Gordon** was blaming the treatment for a whole host of issues and not really taking any responsibility. It's hard to tell a cancer survivor that he needs to get off the couch, but I have to often. Wallowing in the "woe is me mentality" is draining and further enhances the debilitation.

So I literally take this one step at a time. My prescription is for 15 minutes of walking, A.M. and P.M, even in hot weather most can do that. I encourage hydration, and then we move to ten minutes of lifting weights. Yes, I sound like a trainer, but these are such simple, easily attainable goals that can have a real life-changing effect. We will check Gordon's results in three months—not wait a year again. Hopefully the energy will be self-propagating. Holistic: that's how we roll!

MR. MILTON

"How long is this going to go on?"

It's the daughter from out of state. Her father is profoundly ill. Yes, he will die from his cancer (pancreatic), but the time line is unclear because he was just diagnosed. Unfortunately, his wife died a few years ago, and he has been living alone. The daughter has to go back to work and cannot take time off to "babysit."

Sometimes I want to say, "Well, if you think life can be inconvenient, what about death!" Of course, thank God I have more self-control than that, whew!

The real problem is not the daughter. She is reacting to the shock and grief, and I am human enough to know that. The real issue is that companies have no room in the schedule for this. There is family leave that people apply for, but so often people are in marginal jobs with this economy and there isn't a lot of tolerance. Even getting more than two to three days off for a family funeral is tough. What do you do when the house needs to be cared for after the funeral? It's enough to make me yearn for the days of communal or at least extended family living. People need to consider when they move away what this means. Just to retire to the sun may not be an option for everyone, especially when one spouse dies, leaving the other alone.

For me, I told my children to put me in an independent or assisted living place, to get help with care. My recommendation is to look into long-term care insurance. Another daughter told me she was irate at her mother for collecting so much and never downsizing, leaving her to clean out the garage and attic. She called it unfair. Again, today I spoke with a different family and advised a facility placement just so that their father isn't home to interfere with the cleaning out process. As seniors, we need to respect our children's time and lives. Get things in order, consolidate bank accounts, pay bills, and don't leave them in debt. Make our lives smaller; it's not about us.

It's not the children being selfish at the end when they ask, "How much longer?"

Maybe we are selfish if we don't prepare. Even then, there is a lot to do at the end.

Isaac

This is a doozy. The patient comes in released from jail for his all-too-frequent petty crimes. He needs treatment and has Medicaid but no disability or other means to be cared for, so he is essentially living on the street. He manages to get an infection and is thrilled to go to the hospital where three meals and a clean bed are provided. After all, he is used to the state caring for him and cannot make it on his own. While there, **Isaac** finds a way to "con" the docs into extending his stay with all sorts of complaints and vague symptoms (weakness, confusion, pain—you name it). He ultimately racks up over $100,000 worth of testing, etc. while in the hospital. He could have rented an apartment and bought food and transport for a few years if we just paid him that much to stay out of trouble. This goes on more than we think.

So he is now discharged, and his living circumstances haven't changed in spite of all the money spent. Ridiculous. We need facilities other than hospitals and jail. We pay in the end anyway. Why not provide?

CHARLEY

"Well, **Charley** it looks like that big tumor is gone. Your pet scan is negative. It's great news. Now you know why we tortured you with the chemo and radiation. Plus since you lost weight, you are now off your blood pressure meds and no longer diabetic, a bonus!"

How could I know this is not the result he wants? Really. After the exam and review of the testing, he says, "Ya know, Doc, now my problem is not the cancer. My wife of 42 years wants a divorce. Guess she could not handle my cancer. How do you like that?"

I tell patients that it is frequently terrifying for the spouse to watch their loved one go through the trauma of therapy. Charley's issues are multiple now. They have to sell their house. He will have to pay her alimony since she does not work. He is ready for retirement, but all of his nest egg is too little for two households now. He is devastated emotionally and financially.

He says, "I was actually hoping the cancer was back. I would not have had therapy, and I would not have had to deal with this anymore."

So sad. Maybe the cancer treatment process kept a couple together that was breaking up anyway. Maybe it's the fear. Certainly some marriages break because one does not want to be left behind so they leave first. Of course it's not just cancer. What happened to Charley happens to women; sometimes it happens after someone has a stroke or heart surgery. Life is complex enough. Living it with someone just logarithmically increases the complexity. Still, I am sorry that Charley won't enjoy his freedom from disease and treatment. I pray that he will find joy after this drama. I gave him news of hope for life that today he doesn't want to live.

LUCY

Just before I enter the room to see sweet little **Lucy**, a breast cancer patient who has come through months of chemo, a mastectomy, and now radiation, my nurse grabs my arm. "Lucy's in tears. Her husband is leaving her, saying he can't deal with this."

Oh brother. Really? Again? Isn't there a quota on this?

Lucy tries, while blinking back tears, to hide her issue. Since my nurse was her confidant, I will not bring up the discussion unless she does. Getting the information from my staff is very helpful, and although I am compassionate, having the expanded view does help my relationships with patients. I am grateful that patients can confide in them, and I do not take their help for granted. In Lucy's case, I will be just the doc and allow others to have the listening ear for her. Being aware helps with my sensitivity without invading privacy. It does not keep me from thinking I'd like to give him my two cents!

LOLA

Lola is a former "prostitute" who has now given up her life of drugs and alcohol and settled down to marry. The "clean" life, however, does not make her immune from disease, and she now has metastatic cancer. Since she has always been a tough cookie, she is handling the news well. After I review the scans and discuss the chemo and then radiation for palliation, she opens up a little.

Lola says, "Doc, I always knew I would die young. Never could have guessed this way."

I just quietly say, "How about we just live for now and let the dying come later. Enjoy that new husband of yours."

She says that he's worried they won't be able to have sex. I say that there is no hindrance, and she asks me to write that down for him. So she leaves with a prescription for "intercourse permitted."

TONY

We manage many patients in their 80s and 90s. (My most senior was 112!) This group has lived through so much that nothing surprises them. They are not shocked or insulted that they have a disease; nor are they fearful or tearful. There is a quiet acceptance that is calming for the rest of us and a lesson here as well. Frequently they bring humor. Actually very few are curmudgeons.

Today **Tony** comes in for head and neck cancer treatment, sure to further affect his swallowing function. It has already resulted in dramatic weight loss. He did not seek attention until one of his children from out of state visited and found him so frail. Today he weighs 94 lbs, down from 105. He is 6 ft tall! We had a feeding tube placed and hope he will gain some weight before therapy.

When we talked about the possible treatments and if he wanted to proceed, he says, "Only if I get half off! After all, there is only half of me now. I ain't payin for the other half that got away!"

I say, "How about we just send the other half the bill when we are done?" That sounds good to him!

NADINE

A patient died this morning. She was joy-filled, giggly, exuberant, meeting challenges like an arm that did not work anymore and recurrent cancer that she battled valiantly for almost ten years. She was just getting to middle age with a young daughter and lucky to have a loving, supportive husband.

Where is today's conversation? It's with another doc. He called to tell me of her passing. She was truly a favorite. We spent some time on the phone remembering her, discussing her spirit more than her case. It helped us both to cope with this sudden event. There is a long story to **Nadine's** case and personal tragedies she faced other than cancer. Today, however, is a day to take her spirit and try to give her strength to my other patients, reserving just a little for me and the other caregivers.

PAULA

Paula looks like a 12-year-old, but she is in her 40s. Not only is she petite, but her mind never had the chance to mature. It's therefore even more tragic to have to show her sister the films depicting new lesions in her brain. She smiles at me, not sure what I am saying. She is cooperative, sweet, and so naïve, maybe God's blessing. This is all so new. A large, neglected tumor is found, and it's made its way through the blood stream to the brain, threatening her life at this moment.

Some cases we cannot get on top of. It's shocking just how fierce the cancer can be. But that is not why I am writing this now. The conversation has to do with the younger sister. I ask her where the patient lives. She said she is with her parents but that her father is disabled and her mother is very ill. This sister has two children of her own to care for. She looks strong, but I see the weariness in her eyes. It stops me. I have nothing to say. The weight is too much. I am as gentle as I can be. I am inspired by her fortitude, and I remember sometimes all that we can do is put one foot in front of another. I think I see the steel-like spine bend just a little as she goes down the hall.

GRUFF AND TUFF

Gruff and Tuff, that's my name for him. It could also be Big and Blustery. Why is it people think they can control everything? Well, if you have been a success, this cancer thing has no frame of reference for you. It can be humbling, but sometimes it's just a pain in the ass. This guy has no time for it, yet since it started in the throat, he only has 50% chance of a cure even with aggressive treatment. It's going to be toxic. He won't be able to swallow; he will need a feeding tube; he will lose muscle mass; he will be brought to his knees.

Right now, I don't say any of this. I just say that I promise to help him and that I have every faith that a strong man like him will be up for the battle. It is a tacit agreement that I won't steal his vigor.

ALAN

Alan is a docile, sweet character who has had success in life and still works. He has a difficult disease that requires chemo and radiation and is unresectable. He is not the problem. Alan has three daughters. They descended on him from around the country. They whisked him away for several opinions and now are all back for the start of treatment. They call the doctors, the offices, there is a flurry of anticipation, excitement, demands, and frankly they are just carrying on with everyone. They've found a way to alienate so many that they don't have faith in anyone. I have to start a new process here and try to get some control for Alan's sake.

After the first treatment and the rounds of intense questioning, hands clasped on knees, leaning forward, on edge, I look at Alan. I say, "Whatever has happened up until now (3 months into the process), ends now. Today we start the actual treatment. It is a new chapter. No more evaluation, investigation, or searching. Today is the first day, and we are in control. Let's begin the process."

I am happy to answer questions along the way, but someone needs control of this rodeo. Families occasionally feel that the whirlwind and drama are their way of contributing to the treatment and may not appreciate that it can interfere instead. When things and people are out of control, it helps everyone if there is discipline and direction. I hope for Alan, the family and my staff that it lasts longer than a few days!

DWIGHT

Dwight is a very proper, hat-in-hand, very elderly man. Yes, there are suspenders, a pocket handkerchief, and a bow tie. He has a sweet smile and bright blue eyes. He is very hard of hearing, so unless I "yell," I don't get any recognition even with the hearing aids. The "children" have flown in from other states to see him. He lives alone and is almost 100!

They have not seen him for four months and so are very surprised by the rapid growth of the tumors on his head. They are skin cancer. He is very fair, and a small dime-sized lesion has grown and spread until now under his hat he is hiding three very large, egg-sized masses. They are not causing him any trouble—no bleeding or pain.

Now starts the tough discussion. The "kids" are due to travel home, and this is very inconvenient, especially if we choose to treat this. We go back and forth for an hour over a decision. They do not want to create a problem since he has no symptoms. It will be hard to get him here daily for therapy, and there is no one to check on him if he needs wound care. I offer to find a doc near to them or see if there is another sibling who can take him home with them- they just look at me. I guess that is not an option. Okay, we can arrange transport but is this man really going to get in a van or bus by himself? Finally I pull him into the essentially soundproof room and speak directly to him. I tell him that the tumors are growing faster than he is aging. I think that is a kind and considerate way of saying, "You may not die before these cause a lot more trouble." And so it is wise to treat him, which of course is what the family wonders. I offer to see him in another few weeks when another relative is coming in for another brief visit. Then maybe we will see the tempo of the growth. It's a tough problem. At some point, we cannot live alone without any care. We all will need help I think by the time you are 100, it's the least you deserve.

ALICE

Alice is mentally challenged. She has a breast cancer that fills her breast and has traveled to her brain. Her smile is large and bright, but the pain in her eyes is the real message. It is impossible to treat everything at once. She is only in her 30s. We start with the brain, start hormone therapy then we will try to control the pain in the breast with radiation treatment. Her insurance is not easy, and no one will give them the pain medications she needs, so they pay out of a very shallow pocket for it.

I say "they" because this story is not about Alice. Her older sister is with her every day. I am amazed that again for another patient, I am seeing this same dynamic. Her eyes are puffy from the tears, stress, and worry. Alice, who is the challenged patient, has actually been the caretaker for her two invalid parents (Yes, this is another case!). The sister has her own children. Now with Alice needing so much care, the sister is in charge of everyone and still working to support her own children. I marvel at her strength, courage, and determination to do all she can for Alice.

Today she went "all over town" to find a place that had her prescriptions. Alice just smiled, but I saw her fatigue. I am overwhelmed by their situation. The sister takes care of the children, goes to the parents and gets them fed and up for the day, and then goes to work. When she comes home, she picks up the kids from school, takes care of the parents, and then packs up Alice in her wheelchair and brings her for treatment every day. Then she heads home to make a dinner for everyone. The problem is that the parents and Alice will further deteriorate, and I do not see where there is any resource of energy, time, or money that is not already spent. Through it all, she is grieving over her little sister's near demise. How can this be this way? All that I can say is, "Let us just take one day at a time." A trite phrase, but what else is there?

OLIVIA

Since there are over 8 million breast cancer survivors, breast cancer consumes a good deal of my practice. You likely have noticed by now how many of these stories involve that diagnosis, either primary or metastatic. **Olivia** wears her ball cap with the shiny pink breast cancer logo. She tries to look bright and in control. A little fuzz is finally coming in after the chemo, and the radiation is causing fatigue. She is off to work after treatment, but today I catch her sobbing in the dressing room.

I ask, "How can I help?"

She says, "Oh, Doc, it's not this. It's everything else!"

How often do I hear that?! Olivia is in her 40s, a single mom, trying to be strong. While she is fighting her battle, her son is fighting his. He fell in with others and was arrested last night for drugs. He also took her narcotics to sell on the street, her sweet 18-year-old son, due to graduate high school and start at community college. Her hope to live long enough to see him get on his feet so he can manage without her has just been smashed. UGH!

MACY

Macy comes for her cancer treatment with her son. He is either on something or challenged in some way I cannot figure out in the short conversations. But he dutifully gets her here every day. She is a dream to treat, but there is another dynamic. An older, controlling, high-powered brother is constantly on the phone with him and checking on all of us. He lives in another state, and I hear him barking in the phone. When I see the patient and son, the cell phone has to be on speaker. I don't mind this a few times, but it is now every day. This over- management from afar is chaotic. You would think as the doc that I could get this under control, but it's probably a dynamic that has gone on long before she had cancer. No matter what I say, it continues. It is interfering with my care of the patient.

Bottom line: there are no rules for managing parents and family with cancer. All of the interplay of personalities and stresses are heightened during this time. I just need to get out of the way. Today I told Macy's son who is here with her that she is dying and nothing we do will stop that. Sometimes stating the obvious helps shake family out of the denial. I hope the son on the phone will come to give love and support instead of control and demands. These two are in real need.

LEE

Lee is a very tiny, 4'9" Asian lady. She is a bundle of energy. We treat her for a cancer that has traveled to her lungs, and she has done very well. Her husband married her when stationed overseas, and they make a comical couple. She is noisy and nosy. He is quiet and is smiling and looks bemused by it all. The adorable thing about Lee is that she wants to share what she knows. So she comes in every day with some little idea or gadget, a poem, a prayer. My office and the department is filling up with Lee. Maybe that's what she had in mind. We fuss over her newest presentation. But I know the attention we pay to her for her daily joys helps to distract from the real reason she has to show up for radiation every day. I am grateful for the distraction she provides to us as well.

JEFF

Be nice to your siblings. **Jeff** and Jane must have really gone "at it" in their time. He now has lung cancer ("I told you so!"), and his sister Jane has moved in since he has no children and divorced his wife many years ago. I can only imagine the discussions at home, because in the radiation department she is always raising holy cane with him. Jeff can hold his own, but she has the upper hand. Jane is diligent with his appointments, manages his medications, helps control his symptoms, and is a great communicator on his behalf. I am a little afraid of her. But she is a reminder that you never know who will come to your aid. So if you are fortunate to have siblings show them some love!

LOUIE

Louie came in for his treatment and was not his usual, jovial self. He shuffled his feet back to the exam room with his head down. When we settled in, I asked how he was getting along here.

He said, "Doc, here I am fine," and then gave a heavy sigh.

So often the outside world interferes, and cancer is the least of the problem. Louie told me that after church his daughter, who is in her 40s, came home, collapsed into a coma, and died—no known reason. She left six children and several grandchildren. Louie's wife died some years ago, so there is no one for him to lean on. The burden of her big family without the children's own father around fell to him. Many of the children were still living at home with her, and she worked hard for their care.

It was difficult to find the words or the blessing in this. I told him that we would do all we could to help him with his cancer because he now had so much responsibility (this late in his life). They were all blessed because he saw his role as working to get them all on their own feet. Behind the sorrow, I could see his focused determination. His need and desire to live was enormous, but the burden was as well. I hoped that his many reasons to live outweighed the tumor cells' attack and that his internal fortitude would heal him and his family.

MATTHEW

I have seen some dramatic, massive cancers growing out from the skin—especially in men, many of whom are very reluctant to look for and accept care. This one in **Matthew** was different because of the location. Frequently, I see a mass over the shoulder on top of the head—sun exposed areas. Not infrequently, I see them in the ear—and several entirely replacing the ear!

Matthew presents with a truly awful problem. Cancer smells, so there is that, but it also deforms. These tumors are like tennis balls coming out from his head with one on either side or close to the eye. The misery is profound for him. Unfortunately, his lack of insurance and what free care doctors and hospitals were able to give have left him with what looks like an insurmountable situation. He even states he thought of "blowing his head off!"

We develop a plan including chemo and radiation, and thank goodness, he responds beautifully. There is some torment, and he needs surgery and wound care, but the power of our tools became visibly evident while he underwent treatment. Matthew will ultimately die from all of this, but he again demonstrates the power of human courage. Giving him treatment everyday also gave him hope. Sometimes just someone caring helps a patient show up for therapy. Not being alone is profoundly healing.

ELSIE

Elsie is terrified. It doesn't help that she has a mental illness. It is difficult for her to fully comprehend a plan for treatment. Every day we need to reinforce with her. She thinks the awful tumor, worse from neglect, is from the treatment. It takes enormous patience in a busy clinic to stop and understand where she is coming from, sit her down, and re-explain—with full knowledge that the words will not last long and we will be right there again tomorrow. You hope that care, explanations, teaching, directions and management can all move the process forward. It is so very difficult for patients who are stuck, and it is so important to be sensitive to their needs.

Life is not linear; it is multifaceted. In medical school, they had just started an ethics committee and class for the students. One major takeaway for me was to remember that everyone comes to a situation with their own value system. I would broaden that to their own psyche, history, emotions, experiences, fears, fortitude, plans, dreams, etc., etc. It is imperative to respect all of this in managing patients with complex issues. We are treating them—not ourselves. It is easy to lose sight. We can be very matter-of-fact about this entire healthcare process, but in truth the patient's perspective is all that matters!

MARTY

Chocolate chip cookies. We serve them with coffee, tea, and nutritional supplements in the lobby. Patients coming for therapy enjoy the environment. They can do puzzles and frequently get so involved that they stay long after their therapy is over. The TV is on; other people are coming and going. It is a very pleasant space.

Marty comes for therapy in a van provided by her insurance company—a nice perk since she has no other way of getting here, being elderly and living alone. One day she tells me that it can be difficult because they "forget her" in spite of our calling to tell them to pick her up. Another day they left her here for 3 hours!

She said, "I don't mind. I ate the cookies, had some tea and milk, and watched people go by. I don't get to do that at the mall anymore."

Marty was making the most of her situation, no complaints or whining. She was just grateful that even when someone else forgot her, "God was providing for her" with the help from others. I told my staff to never run out of the cookies; we may not appreciate all they provide!

TEAM

My biggest pet peeve. I called another office and heard: "The girl who sched-
ules that is off today." Okay, some days I blow my stack! No, it is not okay to
tell patients about a "glitch" in the office. Just have someone who is there taking care of it. I have a short fuse for messages like that.

How about getting a message like, "I'm away from my desk or on another
line, etc., etc., etc." WHO cares?! Just say leave a message and I promise to call.
Especially for a patient with cancer. We are not ordering shoes or making hair
appointments. This is serious stuff. The staff in any medical office needs to appreciate that a call from a patient is a lifeline. They need attention, immediate
if possible, not because they are in crisis but because it's the right thing to do.

An employee manager from another company once told me, "Oh, Doc,
we can't answer the phone at our offices. We get too many calls!" So everything
goes to a voice mail box. Obviously I am not a fan of phone trees for a medical
office. Hope that manager does not get cancer and have to wait to hear from
the doctor. That is not management or patient care.

There is an office that if you call and they "deem your message not to be
medically related, you will be charged $25." That takes the cake! It's downright
hostile. Managing the staff is managing the patients. Training them to pick
up, triage the call, and help the patient now is a culture. I am happy to say my
staff "gets it," and it makes them happier to work here because everyone is on
the same page and we are all proud of our team approach. Respect for each
other and all of our patients is a culture worth enforcing.

EMMA

After knowledge, docs need patience! **Emma** is a middle-aged woman with breast cancer. I am asked to see her about disease in the brain. In the intake portion of the consult, I find that she had a tumor the size of a baseball in the breast when she finally got medical help. Now it's in her bones, brain, and lungs. I ask her what was going on that she did not get attention sooner.

She answers, "I was scared."

She tells me it was her fault—something I do not like to hear because we can't rectify history and guilt has no part here. But I need to know what she was thinking at the time and then just move forward. Now she wants to be cured (of course!). I realize that fear is a major part of the disease that I have to help control. Laying out a plan, being deliberate and focused, giving her tasks, giving her hope will get her on track. Since her family and husband are with her, I wonder if her words are more for them as an apology. I am biting my tongue—after all, you realize, I am human too.

I want to claim *"It's too far along!"*

My mother would say, "That's not nice, Joanne."

I feel helpless because we cannot rescue her now. The only thing I can offer is that while we work through the treatment, I help her to forgive herself while I avoid judgment and have supreme patience. Doctors have to remember: we cannot treat or rescue everyone from themselves. We can just be available when they finally decide that they want help. And remember to be gracious always. Mom's voice in my head.

ORLANDO

This is clever. The very "active" prostate patient, **Orlando**, has such a big prostate that he cannot urinate. Short anatomy lesson: the urethra travels through the center of the gland coming from the bladder to the penis. It's as if the prostate is in the way for some men with hypertrophy (BPH) or cancer. So the doctor sent him for radiation therapy for the cancer, but so far it is not helping the urination due to swelling.

He comes in for treatment quite disgruntled. The urine may be flowing, but the catheter is a big problem. "Doc, how am I supposed to have sex?!" He is completely shocked by the turn of events.

So I call the urologist, and he changes the catheter to suprapubic (coming out of the abdomen from the bladder to drain the urine, not involving the prostate or genitals.) He is happy as a clam with his new plumbing, and everything is working properly. Respecting quality of life is important!

TYRONE

Tyrone is a good ole', church going, God-fearing, Southern boy with a hitch in his giddy up. (Yes, I talk this way after visiting with him!)

After his exam today, he said, "Well, Doc, I got me some of them new fangled (yes), long-lasting light bulbs. I bought six of them for over $140!"

I said, "What's so special about them?"

He said, "They predict my life expectancy!"

"Wow," I said. "That's terrific. How exactly does that work?"

"Well, they're supposed to last 20 years, and since I am 81 years old, I figure I gotta live to at least 100 or they have to give me my money back!"

I said, "With your sense of humor, that's an easy prediction."

He said, "Yeah, well you have to make sure that if I die before then that they put the refund money in my coffin!"

I so love a sense of humor!

ARTHUR

Arthur is from war-torn Bosnia. He came to the U.S. for a better life for his children. Just when they were starting their secondary education, he was diagnosed in his 40s with lung cancer. He went through surgery, chemo, and radiation.

He said, "I will do whatever it takes to see my children educated here. Please help me survive."

Eighteen months after his diagnosis, the cancer came back, and he was re-treated with chemo and radiation. Today he is here, two years later, with a "clean" scan, looking fantastic and with great energy and a positive attitude. I reviewed his scan in detail and advised him of the great report.

He said, "Doc, I have a confession. You know how I go home to Bosnia every summer to see family? Well, I am also seeing a 90-year-old man who inspires me. I met this man in a village where they believe he has experienced a miracle. The man was told 40 years ago that he had leukemia after he had been treated for another cancer. There was no treatment. He did a favor for a young single mother, helping with her house, and she was very grateful. The woman told him she was a pharmacist and that since he would not accept payment and she knew of his problem, she would give him a gift. That gift was a special tonic with eleven ingredients which are still a secret. It formed a black liquid. The elderly man took the liquid, and when he was examined by his doctor, he was found to be free of his leukemia."

My patient had gone to see him and was gifted with the tonic.

He said, "Doc, this is what is keeping me cancer free. Every year I visit that man, and he gives me hope."

He is convinced that this magic liquid has cured him also. Who am I to say otherwise? Someone even with a strong immune system would rarely survive metastatic lung cancer. Of course, we don't know how long this will last, but I am a fan of his visit to Bosnia, believing that inspiration and will to live keep him cancer free. However, I did ask him to try and find out just what is in that tonic! I can guess two ingredients: miracle and hope.

HAROLD

We do not want it to be, but so much of medical care is about the money! **Harold** is young, only 47 and he has metastatic disease. He needs chemotherapy, but the co-pay is $3,000 just for one treatment. He has been out of work for over six months due to surgeries and therapy, so this is an impossible bill to pay. He is torn: knowing he will die from his disease, not wanting to burden his family with his medical bills, caring for his children, having a wife who is his patient advocate and so she misses work for his appointments. It is all just too much.

His wife left the room for a few minutes, and he quietly asked me a question. "Doc, how can I die more quickly? I can't put them all through this. I would do anything for them. It's bad enough knowing that I will die early, but to leave them with another burden is torture."

Now this is unusual, because most patients want to know how we will battle the disease and eke out as much time and quality as possible. For Harold, I need a different plan. I have to come up with the words that will leave them feeling good about the decision and not that they are giving up or missed an opportunity. I need to not let them feel shame about the decision.

I also need to remind them that we do not know how long we have. I do not want to give him false hope that further treatment will prolong his life. Many things happen, like pneumonia, blood clots, infections, hospitalizations, and falls, related indirectly to the cancer which shortens a life even more than the disease itself.

And so the plan? Hospice. "Let others care for you. Lighten the hardship on the family. Enjoy what time you have. Do not spend every living moment under treatment. Let's get you back to being a dad and husband, not a patient. Enough is enough. You've done your work, now stop all the doctors' visits and live."

ALYSON

It's rainin'; it's pourin today. **Alyson** has been under treatment for a few years and is only 39. Most recently she had brain surgery and is here to get the follow-up radiation. Her husband drives her to the appointment. He is a real bully. I have seen him in the past snarling over her appointments or co-pays. My staff has raised their suspicions about him. Today, Alyson presents with a bruise over her cheekbone.

I ask what happens and she says, "Oh it must be from the brain surgery." Duh. Do people just forget I am a physician? The two areas are not related! So I walk her back to the treatment room, sit her down on the table, and just look at her. No accusations, just concern. Alyson starts with a few sobs, mostly out of fear to beg me to ignore this. I tell her I have a responsibility to report abuse if I suspect it. She says she would deny it anyway because if he is arrested (having other violations), there would be no one to care for her young children (3) when she dies.

I caution her that leaving her children in his care is dangerous. I advise her to call a relative to start to get involved even though her husband refuses to allow it, to be honest with them about what is happening and encourage her support system to keep her children together. She will not be able to die in peace unless this is done. I call children and family services and asked them to check regarding my concerns. I give her the name of a family lawyer.

It is so easy to say, "Stop being a victim," but what a challenge for someone who has lived their whole marriage that way. It takes some of her valuable time, but she eventually leaves her home and moves in with a family member, obtains a restraining order, and gets the court involved. When the time comes, I pray that she will be able to go in peace knowing her last work was rescuing her children.

MR. AIMS

Mr. Aims is quite exuberant today. He is here for a routine checkup and has been cancer free from head and neck tonsil cancer for two years. The treatment has caused a significant weight loss, but as he puts it, "I am down to my fightin' weight and did it the hard way."

Mr. Cotton has just gotten started with the exact same diagnosis and management and is terrified. He comes into the office with big doe-eyes, fear written all over his now emaciated face, holding onto his equally terrified wife. The two patients begin to pass in the hallway, and I recognize an opportunity. I ask Mr. Aims if he would mind sharing, and he is more than happy. He enters the room with Mr. Cotton, and I leave them alone for several minutes.

When I check in, the sun is streaming in, Mr. Cotton is smiling for the first time I have seen, the men are vigorously shaking hands, and we all visually see the hope. It's a blessing to us all—serendipity, really—and I remember how the patient can be the doctor.

Ms. Gabby

Ms. Gabby has breast cancer in her liver, bones, and lung and she has been in this battle for years. Today she has new makeup and spunky hair with blingy sandals on her feet. I can tell she is probably a little hyper from the steroids.

As I enter the room, she robustly announces, "Doc, I am going to kill every cancer cell in my body!"

She is nervous today because we are about to look directly at her recent pet scan and see the results of her new biologic therapy.

"I say, Ms. Gabby that is the spirit! And if you don't believe it, then it can never happen."

How she maintains this level of optimism is beyond me. She has been through several rounds of surgery, chemotherapy, and radiation and has lost and grown hair and eyebrows several times over. She has an entire collection of head wraps, hats, and funky wigs—even walkers and canes. Last year she got a tattoo where her right breast had been. We pull up our chairs to the computer station, and I begin to scroll down the scan. I like to review the images before I read the report and then see what the radiologist says. You can guess what happened next. The liver lesions are gone; the lung involvement is absent; the fluid in the lung is minimal; the bones show signs of treatment but only one has activity. In all, her scan is almost normal. The report confirms dramatic results.

We set up a time to treat her one bone finding so she won't have trouble with her golf and tennis game, and she says, "Told ya!" and bounces out the door.

Ms. Gabby thinks she cured her cancer, and once again, I confirm the power of the positive.

MABLE

As I enter the room, there is a frail, elderly woman in a wheelchair next to an equally elderly but fit man, her husband. He has lung cancer, but his main concern is living to take care of his wife. His history intake is minimal, but he is eager to share about Mabel. His diagnosis and symptoms are punctuated by stories of fishing on his boat. As it goes, he and **Mable** love to fish and have enjoyed a quiet, rural Florida life for 53 years of marriage.

One day he noticed a hole developing and decided it was time for a new boat. The day he bought his boat, Mable had a stroke. After some rehab, he was eager to get her out on his new vessel. While in the shallow waters fishing, she had another stroke (affecting the opposite side of her body). Since life is stranger than fiction, and they really loved fishing, once she improved, again they attempted to go out together on the new boat, and when they returned, Mable had a stroke that took her speech.

I agree this is an amazing coincidence, and I wonder what is going on with this new boat. I never do get satisfaction about why these episodes are happening. They both today, however, seem in good spirits. We get back to the issue of treating him, and after the discussion about therapy with chemo and radiation for his lung cancer, Mable has a few questions that she haltingly writes on a pad of paper she carries. Her last comment is heartbreak to me:

"Tell me when he is gonna die so he can take me out on the boat one last time."

Sigh.

CHESTER

Chester arrives in the office with great enthusiasm, clumsily stumbling over his feet, looking every which way and easily distracted. He is in his training vest and harness, but the Labrador puppy has not yet read the memo. The generous couple has requested to bring Chester into the office to train for socialization. He will, after many months, then be handed off to a veteran as a comfort pet. Until then, he needs to learn how to manage in different environments. The patient and his wife have routinely taken on these responsibilities, although it is very hard after attachment to turn their charges over. That takes enormous heart.

Chester becomes part of our unit for six weeks. We watch him grow, and everyone, patients and staff fuss over him. He rolls around on the floor for tummy rubs and lifts the spirits of everyone here. Someday Chester will have a real job with one of our vets, but for now he has gifted all of us with laughter and joy, such a critical part of healing. We miss him already!

HANK

"Too fast and snarky!" said the South Dakota native, now transplanted to Florida.

I said, "Okaayy." I am just beginning to introduce myself and did not have the chance to be fast and snarky yet.

His daughter interjected that **Hank's** last visit with another doc was less than helpful and that they are in my office to get him back on track. I used to speak fast, and it would irritate patients who took me for a big-city person, maybe overly confident and possibly arrogant (Hope not!). I try to tone it down. The new doc from NYC will learn too that the entire goal is to meet the patient where THEY are, not "talking down" to them but watching for their response. If there is no relationship, there will be no treatment or ability to help. Mirror the patient's tempo, respect their explanations, carefully answer their questions, and test for understanding.

It turned out this patient was very well informed and had researched his disease and treatment options, but he would not suffer snarkiness!

MISS GERTRUDE

A word of advice: whatever your relationship "tolerance" is, please check in on your family! I mean lay eyes on them. Fred arrived with his thin, ill, frail mother. It's obvious she did not get into this mess overnight.

I ask **Miss Gertrude**, "When did you start to notice a change?"

She tells me about three years before. She now has an incurable, life-draining lung cancer. She has lost 80 lbs in 2 years. Fred is here to save the day, pressuring for treatment and cure now.

I ask him, since he just arrived from Chicago, how she had been six months prior at Christmas and who saw her.

"Well, my sister lives here, so I thought she was taking care of her." Fred took a leave from his "important job," and left his wife and kids in Chicago to "take care of this." I understand Fred's disappointment. He seems incredulous. To my point, too often estrangement just leads to strange—because family members are still responsible for each other. Do yourself a favor; see them now, even if it's only for your own benefit. It may save heartache and drama down the road.

MARGARET

"I don't want treatment; my daughter dragged me in here! Everyone dies anyway!"
I'd heard **Margaret** was resistant to care from the referring doc.
"I don't want to get on the table; I don't want to be examined."
Essentially, "Leave me alone to die."

By asking simple questions, not pushing, and redirecting the dialog, I get her to calm down. Often I see patients who would rather die quickly than inconvenience their family. After an hour, I get to the bottom of it, and this one is an eye opener. Margaret lives in assisted living due to a minor, non-cancer related issue.

In her frustration, she says, "Why bother doing anything? When you get old, everyone dies. They just get more frail and old. Why extend that?!"

Margaret is in her 70s and is actually fit and energetic. She is also terrified about what she sees daily, which has impacted her perspective on senior living. I am able to explain that if she lived in an active community, she would see value to living well and at least consider therapy.

Margaret seems in disbelief with this perspective, and now her daughter realizes why her resistance was so profound. She is going to move her mother to a more appropriate setting for active adults.

It was a delight to participate in the "ah-ha" moment for both of them. And so we developed a plan of care for the healthy, hopeful Margaret.

"App"-titude

Why can't a patient with cancer just deal with their own life, death, and issues for once? Why does it seem everything else in life just piles on at the same time? We live our lives one day, one year, one graduation, one marriage, and (usually) one job at a time. Linear is ingrained. So here we are with a new event, one that is life threatening, terrifying, and physically, emotionally, and psychologically altering, but we have to just "fit it in." It's like getting mugged and battling the attacker while your car is rolling down the hill. Or maybe you can't use the stun gun because your arthritic hand can't put enough pressure on the button or your phone is playing a bright, Caribbean ring tone reminding you to pick up your son from ball practice. REALLY, can't we just have one issue at a time, please?

They say this "new" habit of multitasking is unhealthy, that it keeps us from accomplishing as much as we hope and destroys our concentration making us less effective, etc. etc., However, suddenly with cancer , our lives are going on and we are watching from above like an out-of-body experience. There is no opportunity for reflection or breathing. You have to get the scan, the porta cath, the chemo, simulated for radiation, see the surgeon, oh and tell your boss you won't be in—maybe ever!

It's no wonder a cancer diagnosis is so traumatic. There is no space in which it "fits." We don't allow ourselves a minute of "extra" time in a normal day "just in case I have to deal with a life-altering problem."

So how do I approach this part of the discussion with patients? I remind them of their strength, I recognize and respect their courage, I tell them they did not get into this trouble overnight. There is time to breathe while we move forward. I encourage them to actually try to keep all the balls in the air, which can distract them from the high drama of the disease, and help them ease into what will surely be a new path for them. I don't try to paint a rosy picture. If it's very bad news, I have a "put things in order" talk, if necessary.

My strength, assurance, and calm demeanor and manner help them see that the sky is not falling—today, at least. As cancer specialists, we are blessed because we think we can rescue people, but we are cursed because we sometimes believe that. We want them to drop everything for the treatment—it's very egotistical. It's good that I realize this so as not to rob the patient of the rest of their life. My goal is always to let them have their life and find a way to minimize the impact, devastation, trauma, and plain thievery of a cancer diagnosis.

THE ACCOUNTANT

"Its TAX season!" says the businessman who runs a tax service.

I am trying to advise him that his "new" business is fighting an aggressive cancer. They have been at this diagnosis for a few years, but things have changed and time is short.

"April 15th is just six weeks away!"

They want to start therapy after taxes. For someone who has lived their business life with that time frame, it's like a kid preparing for Christmas. It is a very fixed time, against which the rest of his life plays out. I tell him that people are relying on him for their taxes, but he may not be there to do them. I say that he may want to advise his clients that they need to secure another service. Somehow people think that since they own a business for many years, they are somehow exempt (good word here) from taking time off for themselves.

"Well that is just unacceptable."

I wonder if I should buy into this and expect a miracle just out of his pure desire to survive past April 15th. As Tax Day loomed large, I began to worry for the clients who, unbeknown to them, would suffer the consequence of not having their taxes filed on time. But the writing is now on the wall and each day is a struggle. He will not see another filing, and I must give him sufficient direction and a recommendation to put things in order. I know, it seems like that is not my concern, but his denial will impact many people. Finally, I realize what I always learn, that people must do what they want even, and maybe especially, at the end of life. It is their call. Sad to say, his death preceded April 15th by a week. There are only two things certain in life.

WHITE COAT SYNDROME

There is a new study evaluating how patients want their doctors to look. If you think about all of the docs you have seen, I am sure everyone was quite different. So the study results state that patients want their docs to look professional, which may or may not include a white coat.

Docs are conflicted about the coat due to documented **"white coat syndrome,"** feeling it is archaic, etc. Many want to wear scrubs in the office (when they originally began as a way to remove street clothes for the OR), and now they are available to everyone as street clothes. So the week the article came out, something related happened here. I had a patient who called my office right after I consulted with her to speak with the secretary several times. She saw me for a second opinion and because my office was more convenient, wanted to be treated here but had some issues.

I fit her into my schedule when asked by a doc in the next office before I was headed out to give a lecture. I was wearing a black suit, blouse, heels, and not my lab coat. I actually do believe in dressing professionally and business attire with or without a coat is my style. Turns out the patient wanted to know if I "ever dress like other docs." My secretary was flummoxed. Eventually it became clear that she wanted a doc who dressed more casually and in a lab coat. That is what made her comfortable. As a female doc who started when the field was male-dominated, I do believe that cultural impressions are ingrained, and so I choose to usually wear a white coat at least the first time I meet a patient. It helps them relate to me as their doc, not an office worker or nurse. So I vote for the white coat and am sure to wear it for my anxious patient with every encounter since she decided to give me another try!

THE WIFE

"Doc I want my husband to live another 10 to 20 years. We can't give up!"

But this patient is challenged with one of the most aggressive cancers and has already lived four years with it. We are at the end of the road, and we can all feel the desperation. I think the patient is at peace, but his **wife** is tearful, begging and bargaining. No attempt by me to "prepare" her is accepted.

Sometimes in oncology we rudely remark that some docs are guilty of treating patients at the funeral home. This means treating until the bitter end. It's not their fault. Some families and patients demand an ongoing, fight-to-the-death plan. Since we generally know a time frame, and here is a patient that has defied all odds, is it unreasonable for him or his wife to assume he still can survive for some time? Well, we are not trying to line up the funeral before its time, but there are cases of patients' families keeping someone on a respirator long after the spirit has left the body. This can give people time to handle the grief, but I am not disposed to encourage Pollyanna thinking.

"We will continue to do what we can," is the best I can offer.

I believe that "words are things," and so some folks think if you say they are dying out loud, it makes it happen. Sometimes even I wonder why it is necessary to bother trying to prepare for the end. After all, when it does happen, they will have to deal, and the grief will be no less. So today my plan is to prepare for the worst but hope for the best and learn a lesson from this man's wife who won't let go.

KOREA

I have three patients (one woman and two men) from Korea now. I mention their nationality because it is critical to their care. First, the families do not in any of the cases want their loved ones to know they have cancer. There are several PhD's in all the children combined. There is lots of note taking, questioning, scan reviewing, and intense conversation, and I am grateful for their avid interest. They clearly adore and honor their parents.

Each patient has metastatic cancer from the lung to the brain—a very devastating and life-threatening disease. So what am I noticing about these three? They are amazingly stoic—always smiling, grateful, warm, not complaining even with challenges, compliant with every direction, and obviously people who previously had control in their lives but who are now willing to abdicate to their children. In two of the cases, I placed the patient in hospice over 18 months ago and yet they survive. Is the family nurturing responsible for their longevity?

They have the exact same therapy as others, and yet there must be a cultural difference. It is a joy to be with them through the process, and I may have to postpone my "end of life" discussions for this group as a whole and enjoy observing the dynamics with wonder.

THE SISTER

The patient had been "living" on the street. He went to an ER for pain and was found to have cancer spread to his bones. He arrives for the appointment quite a bit disheveled and dazed. Even more dazed is a family member by his side that had not seen him for years. Over the course of his management, they appeared to have re-bonded and as his pain was managed and he had a "home," his strength, attitude, and sense of wellbeing increased. At one point, he arrived alone, and we learned that his sibling had suffered a stroke.

He then implored me, "Doc, I did not care about anything that happened to me, but now you need to keep me around to care for my **sister**. I am all she has."

His will to live and newfound purpose still sustains him, and he dotes on her, feeds and helps her to walk.

He says, "I just needed a reason to live, and now I know what that is".

JOE

The big, burly ship's mate lumbers down the hallway with wide eyes and a sweaty brow. **Joe** is terrified. He was treated for lung cancer with chemo and radiation three years ago and is here to review his new pet scan. If all is good, he will sail out for six months. If not, it's back to treatment—no income, lots of drama, and no guarantee.

We look at the scan together, and his relief is so dramatic that he jumps up, hugs my shoulders, and declares, "Thank you, mamma bear!" (Yes, its transference but I don't care.)

I am so relieved for him. But then I sit him down and remind him that belly fat will kill him before the lung cancer and to get serious about it.

He says, "Yes ma'am."

He won't.

Then I ask, "How are you going to live the next six months. It is a torture for you, living between office visits." (There's a great book by Dr. Bernie Siegel on this.)

I have an idea. I ask him to reach in his pocket for change. "Now give me a coin (it's a nickel). Put your initial on it (we found a marker pen), and give it to me. Now I am going to hold onto this for you. This represents your cancer. I have it. I will keep it, and you can be free to let it go and not worry. BUT I have one request: on the next visit, if your scans are still negative, I want a quarter!"

Joe said, "Doc, if I am still disease free, I am gonna look for a half-dollar!"

I said, "What, Joe are you now bribing me?"

I still keep a yearlong desk planner. I taped the nickel on the date of his next visit. As Joe strutted down the hall with a huge grin on his face, I called after him.

"Don't forget to lose some weight!"

He called over his shoulder, "Yes, sir!"

He won't.

Raj

"Namaste!" **Raj** is a gentle, peaceful soul, accepting of his cancer diagnosis and coming to treatment joy-filled, bright, and calm every day.

I ask his wife if he is this happy at home, and she confirms. "Oh, yes, Doctor, he always has been for over 40 years!"

Raj bursts with radiant energy. He tells me that when he awakens, he just cannot wait to get up and going, feeling so joyful and thankful for every moment. He never had a side effect from treatment, never complained, was ever ready to exclaim how strong and powerful he felt, and was always sharing his happiness with the staff and others. When it came time after two months for his therapy to end, I told him how much we would miss his spirit here, but I know he has others who need his force. It was a God-send that he was here at the same time we had several very challenged and challenging patients. I feel that some people are sent here because we need them.

As Raj signed out, my medical assistant rounded the corner with a new patient. I did a double-take because his body habitus—tall, thin, full head of grey hair—was so similar to Raj's. They even had the same diagnosis. The patient told me he passed several centers to come to ours and that he just felt this was where he should be. When we finished the consult and consent, he stood to leave and bowed.

"Namaste."

Aaah, we are good for another two months!

RUTH

Ruth is a hardcore New Yorker who moved to Florida not because all old people should eventually come here, but to have her son help to care for her while being treated. She "hates" it here. (No "Namaste" from Ruth!) She would rather be at home with her mahjong ladies. She is willing to put up with all this fuss but has no delusions of a happy ending to it all. I appreciate that most seniors need help, but many prefer to live in their communities with familiar activities as long as possible. Driving is a big deal—once that is taken away, look out! So many patients live in their children's homes with nothing to do all day and no one to take them to their favorite places while the children work.

Ruth says not to worry about the cancer because she is rapidly dying of boredom.

One day she says, "Doctor Dragun I have to give you something before I die."

I say, "Ruth, you have time. Let's see how the treatment goes."

But she was adamant. The next day she comes with my gift: Ruth hands me a "dammit doll!" What? It says to "grab it by the legs and slam it on a table yelling 'dammit!'"

I have never seen anything like this. It's fabric, stuffed, and frankly not cute. I find it a little creepy, especially because I try to have a peaceful demeanor in the chaos here, so no dammit for me!

Ruth says, "Doc, you never know when you will need it!"

I ask Ruth if she uses one regularly! I think that says it all about how Ruth felt. I see her every time I open the drawer with some precious mementos from my patients, but I haven't found a reason to pull that one out and use it yet!

CHARLIE

Whatever your business, you follow certain rules. In medicine, regulations were made that we need to address patient's pain in an organized and standardized way. A pain scale of 1-10 was developed for routine use in every clinic. Think about pain. When you have it, you don't think, "Well it's only a five." No it's the worst pain because it's all you have at the moment. It could be a toothache, a back spasm, a fractured leg, a paper cut.

After we ask this "profound question" to rate the pain, then docs have to document what we are doing for the pain. In the meantime, there is an opioid epidemic leading to heroin, and prescription pain killers are the culprit. So now we are expected to measure the pain but not to treat it. What a disconnect.

So **Charlie** comes in and says, "Doc, this is by far the worst pain I ever had!" He is young, getting chemo and radiation, and having some side effects that he is poorly tolerating. We are always guarded when we write for narcotics and now we are required to query a government database when we do. Then someone in the government checks to see how often we docs actually do the querying! I guess if I fail, I won't have to treat pain any longer.

A whole taxpayer-funded industry has sprung up! Why? All because we cannot trust physicians who trained for a minimum of ten years to find and manage pain. The government is so much better at it?!

So to investigate this episode further, I ask Charlie some questions. Finally, when he says, "Doc, this is even worse than the pain I had when my friend shot me!" I write the script.

MISS GREEN

"**Miss Green**, what is going on?"

"Well, my sister won't let me sing in the gospel choir!"

I ask if she is having problem with her voice—hoarseness, difficulty swallowing, weakness—and we do the whole system review. I think it's pretty comprehensive, but I am not prepared for this.

"Look at my head, something is growing up there!"

On the top of her scalp, buried in her hair, there are at least two masses. They represent a skin cancer—very treatable but disturbing. They are horny, scaly, protruding and unfortunately on both sides of the scalp. I asked what this had to do with choir singing.

"Well, my sister has pestered me my whole life. When I showed them to her, she said I was growin horns like a devil, and now she is telling everyone about this and they are lookin at me funny and whispering around me."

I advised Miss Green to take a break from the choir for now. I gave these lesions radiation, and they flattened out and disappeared. Unfortunately on the follow-up visit, she had the expected side effect (patchy alopecia) and a bald spot from the radiation right in the middle of her head. I asked if she had gotten back to singing.

She said, "Oh, yes, I did! I told my sister that there was no devil in me because now I am proud and, with this bald spot, lookin like a monk!"

Atta girl!

GERTRUDE

I had some bad news for sweet **Gertrude** today. Just three months after treatment, the cancer is coming back and spreading. It is tough news for this sweet 87-year-old, but she understands that at an advanced age, longevity has already been attained and treatment is now a quality of life issue—in other words, just treat if it keeps her from being ill (bleeding, pain, etc.), not to prolong her life.

Her main issue isn't the cancer. Her concern is, "Can I still drive the bus?" Gertrude is and has been for over 40 years a school bus driver—even throughout treatment—and you can tell it is a lifeline. The kids, the route, and the parents are all pure joy for her. I am a big fan of keeping life as "normal" as possible, even while the world seems so out of control for patients. I encourage Gertrude to continue working as long as she can (and if she still passes the driver's test).

Before I leave the room and we share a hug, she looks up and says that there is one more thing. She says, "I don't want any treatment that will cost me money. Another reason I work is to bring in some income, and I can't be using it all up and leave nothing for my husband. He is not well, and we both always thought he'd be the first to go. But now, I am the stronger one, and it looks like my time is up. He will need care, and it breaks my heart that I will not be here, so I need to make sure I have left something for him."

Gertrude is ever the caregiver. I assure her that we will comply with her wishes, and she is very relieved getting that off her mind. Recall that in med school ethics we are taught to always look at a situation from a patient's perspective and value system, not our own. In cancer care, we get a lot of practice.

BRIDGETT

Bridgett is by her partner's bedside. The two senior women are both in their late 70s and have been partners for life, having met in high school. The patient is dying; her diagnosis is such a thief. Not only is it taking her life, but also any time to prepare. She is quickly intubated and placed on a ventilator. A cancer diagnosis rarely does this. An accident, a heart attack, a stroke, quick and over, but cancer usually allows for preparation. Not this time.

This is a situation I will never forget. Bridgett sat with the patient for days, almost never leaving her side.

About day four or five, as it appeared there would be no reversing the situation and someone needed to make a decision regarding the "tubes," the patient's family began to come in—sisters, a brother, a nephew. When they arrived, Bridgett's visits were interrupted. Once when she stepped out, she found me in the hall and asked to discuss the situation. I thought it would be about the intubation and timing. Instead it was more info about their relationship. She told me the family had never approved and blamed her for keeping their sister from having a "normal life." They do not speak to her and they did not spend holidays together, essentially abandoning their sister. Now at the end, they are called to be involved as "next of kin" because there is no paperwork to suggest otherwise.

When Bridgett had gone home the day before, the house had been cleaned out by the "family," and she was told she needed to vacate. Cold. I am sickened, even now when I remember this time. It leads me to discuss end of life and preparations with patients' family and especially for the unofficial partners (men and women). I am certain Bridgett's partner would have prepared for this exit. Now she has no one, and I am truly saddened for her and hope that my encouragement to families and patients to prepare will spare heartbreak for others.

THOMAS

Thomas is in his 80s. I think that is the average age of my patients, not a surprise since the expectation is that cancer will afflict one in two or three people as seniors live longer. We have to get more creative in how we manage people with multiple co-morbidities. It is not unusual to have multiple cancers, heart disease, diabetes, and a stroke. Many issues confound our immediate care plan. For Thomas, he had prostate cancer and now has a different cancer requiring chemo and radiation. It's a tough plan, but he looks able to manage and has great family support. He is proud to wear a hat stating he is a Korean and Vietnam War veteran.

In a military town with a naval air station, I am honored to care for many veterans. My father was in Patton's Army, and my husband was in the Army Corps of Engineers in Vietnam.

Thomas is only ten days into treatment when he becomes profoundly weak after his first chemotherapy. His issue is that he has nocturia—up several times during the night to urinate because of the prostate history. One night, he takes a bad tumble and ends up in the hospital for several weeks and then rehab for fractures, weakness, and significant cardiac issues. When he came back to see me, the contusions on the face are still evident.

Of course, he quickly said, "You should see the other guy!"

We chuckle at how he survived two foreign wars with several deployments but barely survived getting up to "pee." We both agree it is time for a bedside urinal, and his wife offers to tuck him in to keep him safe. A hero in life, Thomas is refusing to have an incidental death.

SONNY

Such a big smile and personality for the elderly man not more than 5'3". When I first meet him, **Sonny** conjures vague remembrance of a performer long ago. Then it hits me, he has the demeanor (not the "schnozzle") of Jimmy Durante (cha-cha-cha) and the tilted hat to boot. Turns out Sonny was a song and dance man and certainly still maintains the charisma. His eyes smile. He knows he is in trouble but hopes something can help. We give him a high dose in just five treatments of stereotactic radiation which targets the tumor and limits dose to normal tissue. It is highly effective for Sonny, and the tumor goes away. He can still sing and smile, but I am concerned.

When we get another scan a few months later, the area we treated is gone, but a new tumor formed and the light is gone from his eyes. I believe at some point the body is overwhelmed, even when a tumor is small. Like Jimmy said, *"Why can't everybody leave everybody the hell alone?"*. I decide that we will leave Sonny alone. Often with doctors, hospitals, and medicine, the opposite happens. *"Everybody wants ta get inta da act!"* I advise Sonny to avoid healthcare because it could be dangerous to his health. He and his family agree. *"That's the conditions that prevail."*

Okay, I'm done.

MARYANN

MaryAnn assures me that she is NOT a hypochondriac! But…

Aah, there it is. I am a good listener and have great empathy for my patients, and so often I realize it's not exactly the cancer or the new little bump or the mole or the swelling. Instead it's anxiety. They just don't know what to fear, but they are sure it's something. Many are hyper-vigilant because a tumor was "missed" or found too late to cure, and now everything is suspect.

I don't blame MaryAnn. She was young when first diagnosed and so has every right to any concerns. I can dismiss 99% of them, and that helps her cope. I have the hardest time keeping her fears at bay for long. Something always creeps in and friends, relatives, and even co-workers just pile on. Everybody has a story, and she sees these as real threats. We often refer patients to therapists to manage their fears or even medicate them with better living through chemistry. The habit of fear and worry needs to be replaced. There is a brain circuit firing all the time, and patients spiral downward even when things are fine.

I do not have any magic. They can read books on brain power, self-help, anxiety, etc., but few are willing to break out of it. So I routinely make a contract with them. It involves exercise. If you just tell a patient to exercise, they won't. It's like telling a smoker to stop—not happening. So I give them very explicit directions. They must start walking for ten minutes A.M. and P.M. ("Doc, it's too hot. Maybe I should do the treadmill;" "I have to pick up my kids;" "My knees hurt;" "I get dizzy.") I've heard it all. I insist they do it and work up to 30 minutes twice a day and document it. No, we don't need the monitoring bracelets and watches. Some are so challenged, I have them count 100 steps then turn around. It is well documented that getting outside in nature, eye movement, and blood flow are all beneficial to health, memory, sense of wellbeing, and anxiety. Also I have them keep a written list of concerns. If they have an ache or pain or some other finding, they write it down. At the end of the week, they are to go through the list and cross off whatever is gone.

When they bring the list in, you cannot believe how long they are, but generally we are down to only about five or so items that still need to be addressed. It gives them a "place" to put their fears, they feel more in rather than out of control, and they know I will not dismiss them when I see the list. The patient and I both like that they now have homework.

SASHA

"How adorbs are you?" **Sasha** is grinning ear to ear as I immediately comment on her new hairdo. It is the first time she is wearing a wig, having come for many rounds of therapy for several months, bald or with a covering scarf.

She says, "My sister made this for me!"

What a blessing, and it's truly inspiring how this improves her self-esteem. Sasha almost forgets the wheel chair, the pain, and the fact that she is in her 30s and has metastatic cancer, children for whom to care, and a job that she goes to while "fitting in" the treatments. She is amazingly upbeat and calm; she always finds something to laugh about—not in a denial-four-stages-of-grief way, just her baseline personality. She lifts everyone around her.

Today is her last day of therapy for a while (I hope), and she wanted to look special for it. I pray that the power of her positivity could kick her immune system to control the disease. She hardly got a chance with it—being diagnosed with stage IV just a few months ago. She delights in the "graduation certificate" and says she will frame this so that every day she remembers how strong she is. Sasha doesn't need a certificate; she just needs to keep smiling and look in the mirror. I am so grateful for her sister's efforts with the pixie wig. We all send her off with lots of hugs, and she waves like a Miss America in her wig and wheelchair. Cancer can't mess with Sasha today!

GIL

The petite, soft spoken "girlfriend" (is there a better word for someone in her 70s?) sits at the edge of her chair with balled up tissues in her lap. She has requested a visit with me without her significant other knowing. She whispers that she does not know what to do, now that **Gil** is failing. The brain, lung, and bone lesions are overwhelming a formerly robust, gregarious, loving man who is now abrupt, cranky, and depressed. They have been together since after their spouses died, for about 15 years. She is someone I spoke to early on about having her "ducks in a row" so that she is not out on the street. Her major issue is whether Gil should be in hospice. I advise her that there is still care he can have—further chemo and radiation if he wishes, but hospice may be in his future or at least a palliative care plan for pain.

My problem is that Gil will not take narcotics because he thinks they are a step to heroin. When he attempted marijuana, he was not as "good at smoking as I used to be." They battle quite a bit now, and it is just breaking their hearts. I put a plan together for hospice that I hope will help, because if the pain is managed, it should calm him down. Then I let them both talk about their frustration with the disease and now each other; they are grieving while he is living. They are so sad that their happiness is suffocated by this tragedy.

Gil is glad and hopeful to hear we have come up with a plan. I remind them they are spending a lot of time, effort, and money (all in short supply) with their doctors. They need to let go of the drama and leave it with us.

"Just be the wonderful couple you are. That is all you need to do. You do not need to manage this disease. I cannot write a prescription for your loving relationship."

I offer that they need to reconnect for what time they have and leave the devil at the door. I have to give them permission to pull themselves out of this vortex and stop identifying with the disease. Cancer is greedy. It consumes the body, the mind, and the spirit so often. I say, "Don't give it your love too." They brightened at this idea. I left them alone in the exam room where they had time to weep together. It was a delight to see them holding each other up as they walked into the Florida sunshine.

CAROLYN

The young, beautiful woman no longer looks like a model. After months battling a brutal cancer, she is profoundly yellow with jaundice. Her doting husband is at her side. They are looking for hope and help. She has several children and would love to get back to mothering, but the entire family is consumed with trying to rescue **Carolyn**. Her eyes are vacant with no expectations. The work of caring for her today really isn't to see if we can radiate an area for comfort. This is probably well beyond that. A pain management team is called on, and we all prescribe medications and palliation. This end of life care still looks like a fight for life to the family, but the patient and I know otherwise.

I ask the family to give us a few minutes alone. Carolyn expresses her concern about leaving her children behind. Her grief is for them, not herself, as is true for all parents with illness. She is Catholic and believes in an afterlife, and we talk about how she will always be there. She is in those children, and they have her strength. She asks me to say a prayer with her. Afterwards, I give her something I found for her when her case was first presented. It's a mala—a necklace or bracelet in agate. We talk about how rosary beads were fashioned from this ancient meditation tool. Agate is a "healing stone." Some believe it is associated with releasing fear and stress, encouraging trust and hope. Energetically, the moss agate is considered to give strength. It also represents new beginnings. I tell Carolyn she can pray to God while wearing the mala to remind herself that she is strong and that even at the end there is a new beginning.

SAMANTHA

"Don't go in there. She is on FIRE!"

My staff is protective, but I have to put my big girl doctor pants on and face the drama. **Samantha** is exploding. She is enraged about iatrogenically induced problems (physician-medication caused issues). These frequently occur when our treatments are toxic or there are side effects to medication. These unwanted effects can often be managed by piling on further meds or therapies, and a whirlwind of cyclical "take this then take that" can dizzy even the heartiest. The cancer is bad enough—who needs added issues?

Samantha is enraged, and while each physician has smugly provided one more prescription that should "fix the problem," nothing is working. She is done with all of us. I know this is frustration, but after a significantly angry visit that I am unable to successfully placate, I make other suggestions with over-the-counter remedies. Ultimately, in a few days, the formula works, and the patient is back to baseline. Samantha graciously apologizes to the staff and me for her outbursts, and we all push onward. I remind the staff and myself of that narrow thread so many hold onto. They think if they can just get through this, if they get some sleep, if they don't throw up after chemo, if the scan looks good…So many negotiations. They aren't aware that docs are doing the same thing: If this can work and help the symptoms then they can tolerate that, or if the scan looks good, no more chemo, or looks bad, then another biopsy. It's always a moving target. Just when everything looks "good," we have to prepare for another insult. Some days it's so hard to find relief, but when it happens (even if it's just getting a night's sleep), it can be nirvana.

PRUDENCE

Prudence was an exotic dancer, but now that she is in her 50s, she just "keeps men company!" When she comes for treatment, every single thing she wears is the same bright, sometimes neon color— from the earrings to the sparkly sandals. The clothes are short, tight, and obvious. If Stacey and Clinton from *What Not to Wear* were still chastising and reinventing, someone would have to call for a Prudence makeover. Not me. She is just as she should be and a breath of sunshine that fills the department. People ask in whispers, "Who is that?!" She is a bright, happy, in-your-face crackerjack in 6" heels that no one can ignore. She is a force and worked all through her cancer treatment 'cause, "Somebody got to pay for me to look this good!"

Today the neon orange is also matched by the lipstick. I tell her, "Prudence, you are so fierce; cancer would be scared to come back in that body."

She says, "Lord have mercy, Doc, I love when you talk dirty!"

What is so interesting about this cartoonish character today is that for the first time, she is not alone. With her is her new beau, and he is the patient! I previously treated Ivan but couldn't remember the timing. Turns out Miss Prudence used to wait in the lobby after her therapy to brighten Ivan's life. So a match made in radiation "heaven" lobby. The big, burly, younger-by-15-years man is also cancer free. He looks like the cat that ate the canary with Miss P on his arm, and she is doting and fussing all over him.

I think my words will be prophetic, not because of neon orange, but because the giggles will boost their immune systems. We are all looking forward to their next follow-up visit!

Mrs. Abruzzo

"Doc, we have a problem. **Mrs. Abruzzo** won't get on the table for her first treatment; she is very distressed."

When I see her, she is visibly shaken. I ask what the issue is. Does she need anti-anxiety medication? Does she have claustrophobia, pain, or any further questions about the treatment? No.

"I can't watch TV anymore!" So this is a new one to me. "Have you seen it lately? Have you seen the commercials? They talk about all the side effects to radiation, how sick you get, pain, can't eat, esophagus problems. They say their whole body is ruined, no way can I get on that table today!"

Mrs. Abruzzi has a small lesion in the far outer edge of her lung and will not have any esophagus issue and other than fatigue probably no side effect at all with stereotactic therapy.

She said, "My biggest problem is that I love game shows and after retiring, really got into them. Now, they are gone for me. You can't turn on any channel without the stop smoking message scaring me to death. Hey, I get it. I smoked but quit 20 years ago, and now that I have cancer I don't need them to scare me."

Actually I agree with Mrs. Abruzzo that these messages, while done for shock value and preaching, do little for anyone addicted to quit. I am of the mindset that changes occur through a positive attitude (Thanks Patty Labelle Philly girl!): "I want to be well. I intend to protect my body. I am a force. I am strong and able." It is not achieved through fear and intimidation. Who do they have on their board and advertising committee? Obviously not someone who has faced this directly, or else they would see the negative unpleasant message as destructive, not uplifting and life altering.

And so we come up with a plan that will satisfy Mrs. Abruzzi: she can watch her shows, but when any health "care" message like the drug companies direct marketing or the negative ads about smoking come on, she is to get up and walk. Moving will improve her mind and body, and she can shake off the "demon threats" of the TV.

Later that day, I heard that specific commercial on a TV in another room. I came back to watch it myself and was horrified. Lung cancer is hard enough. It is still the primary cause of cancer death in men and women, and so smoking is terrible, but negative messaging and fear mongering doesn't work for anything. Maybe Mrs. Abruzzo will like walking so much she will turn off the TV and walk right out the door and get some fresh air too. Now there would be a winner!

JEREMY

Medical records are "nosey" for a reason. We've all sat through the "fill out papers and bring with you" lists every office has. Even if you go for a sprained ankle, they want to know your last prostate or mammogram exam. It makes healthcare expensive and inefficient but "complies" with regulations. A major part of the interrogation, however, is family history, most important for cancer care (not a sprain). Even before the mapping of the genome, we knew patterns existed for some cancers: breast, prostate, GI, even lung. Now we can examine blood and determine if there are genetic predispositions. While we are busy doing that, I find the process of asking about family important for many other reasons. Aunt Sally had breast, Uncle Tim prostate, dad lung, and mom uterine etc., etc.

Today when I met **Jeremy**, there was a long list of various cancers on his mother's side, but I was curious how his brother died young. He whispered "murdered." I knew I'd heard right because of his pained voice. How very tragic. He then talked a little about his brother and his own cancer drama disappeared.

The parents are here too, and they say, "Now Jeremy is our only son, and we are terrified for him."

It is the anniversary of his brother's death. There is so much pain in the room; I think the oxygen is gone. There is no way to lighten the moment.

I softly say to his parents, "You have two sons, and I believe your brother sent you to see me today and he is looking out for you. He is giving me a big responsibility and I assure you we will do our best."

Acknowledging this other person in the room seemed a relief to them, and they left still frightened but less burdened. They asked me to pray for them, and I told them that is the most important part of my job.

Justus

The room is a hub of activity—little ones are trying out the stethoscope on a sneaker, looking through the light at their fingers wiggling, the older one blowing up rubber gloves, playing with the plastic model of a prostate—lots going on today! **Justus** is a young man with several children and a brain tumor. His wife works, and so he cares for the children, taking them everywhere. His cancer was treated at a major university hospital three years ago, and he is back to decide if the new scan suggests he needs more therapy. He is very resistant to considering anything that limits his current abilities or takes time away from family.

When I examine Justus today, he still has the flat affect and doesn't look me in the eye. That is his baseline personality, not due to an abnormal brain. He is painfully shy, today, a little scared. I settle the children in chairs and pull the youngest into my lap. We swivel to look at the MRI on the screen that he had performed yesterday. It still shows an abnormality of various shades of grey and white squiggles around a central hole, just beneath the interrupted bone in the skull. No change. I have offered him treatment for recurrence over the past year; the docs have tried to get insurance to pay for temador chemo. Justus and I have an agreement: if the tumor does not show growth, he wants to hold therapy. His exam is excellent—great strength, no numbness, normal gait, no falling over, no vision issues, and all the piercings and tattoos that cover him intact. The kids now have outlasted their attention spans, and chaos takes over.

I am happy for Justus. We both know it's not about him. We will check again in three months. I am beginning to watch these children grow up and hopefully continue for a few more years. He is very relieved today, and when he leaves and they all tug on his pants out the door, he stops, turns, and looks me right in the eye as he softly says, "Thanks, Doc."

PATTY

"I might be pregnant!"

Wait, what? During radiation, women up to age 60 (huh?) get pregnancy tests to ensure it is safe to deliver radiation without affecting an unborn fetus, which could have devastating consequences. **Patty** is young but has a cancer in her bones, and we are giving radiation to her pelvis. Therefore, pregnancy is NOT an option. She and her boyfriend decided that they want to have a baby and so are "working" on it. We have a long, rather dogmatic chat whereby I am insisting she uses a form of birth control, even abstinence. It's just ten days more of treatment. Patty tells me that her boyfriend will not go for that and asks if she can just ignore my advice but get a pregnancy test every day during therapy?! Nu-unh, no way and no how. She is absolutely opposed to any restrictions, mostly out of reluctance to tell her boyfriend.

Bottom line for Patty isn't the pregnancy. It's more complex. Patty craves independence. She doesn't want to be reminded that she has stage IV cancer and be doted on. She doesn't want to see the fear in her family's eyes as she knows that she will not survive this. Her boyfriend said that she can stay with him, but in exchange, he wants to have a baby. I tell her she can be fitted for birth control without hormones (which would work against her cancer), but he is controlling. Patty would be best served by being completely on her own, but that is not in the economic cards.

So for now I offer two options: stop treatment altogether, even though any medications for pain would be toxic to a fetus and therefore also not permitted, or move back with her family for ten days while we do the radiation. I speak to her mother with Patty in the room and advise her that she is to try as best as possible to ignore her cancer. They need to be mother and daughter, not nurse and patient. Her mother understands and is willing to try. I ask them to take a walk together every day and not speak of the cancer for 30 minutes. It will help both if they can re-bond and learn to enjoy each other. A baby is not an option.

MR. CLARK

Mr. Clark is a Korean War Army hero. He has a very heavy New York accent but migrated to Florida 40 years ago (he is 87!).

I say, "Really, Mr. Clark this treatment won't help extend your life. It's a small tumor and not causing any problems, so why come all the way across town in traffic by yourself and risk side effects that may be worse than the cancer?"

He tells me that he feels great and fully expects to live to at least 100 so he wants to do all that he can. I agree now since small-field stereotactic radiation should be well tolerated. That is not the real story. When he came for treatment, he arranged his own transportation with the V.A. He is legally blind, hard of hearing and stands 5'2" but is even shorter due to the hunched spine and use of the walker.

He says, "Doc! This tumor won't kill me, but the bus service will. I was on hold for a full 45 minutes to make arrangements. They kept telling me to submit forms I already sent, passed me around, dropped the call, and had me explain over and over. It took me three hours to line up a 20 minute trip. I should a' taken a friggin' pill to calm down before I called!" A man can survive the Korean War, live a full life for 87 years, run a successful company, still be tough as nails, and have every intention to never give up and live to 100, but the V.A. inefficiencies take him down. Please help us take better care of our veterans.

P.S.: The treatment worked, and he has no side effects and is disease free.

Molly

Molly smoked for 50 years, starting at age 11, so no surprise about the lung cancer. She is determined to beat this, and as I have always said, it's not usually fear of dying that gives a person the momentum to fight. After all the plans are made for treatment, she asks if it can hold for another two weeks. I am thinking it's summer and she may have visitors and take vacation first. When she returns, everything goes smoothly and she has minimal side effects and since she is a widow, transports herself. As we get more acquainted, I ask if she has any family in the area.

She hesitates, but then with a sigh tells her story. Her son's wife died of cancer, and they have two children. After her daughter-in-law's death, her son began drinking and was unable to care for the children. Rather than have them taken by the state, Molly took them in with her. The granddaughter is ten and the grandson thirteen. Sophie is strong and healthy, but Daniel is severely handicapped. He goes to a boarding school during the year, but Molly cares for him in the summer, hence the need to postpone treatment.

"So, you see, Doc, it's not about me." She is trying to get her son involved in the event she can no longer care for them. She thinks it was the stress that took her daughter-in-law. By the time her treatments have finished with me in October, her son is making supervised visits with the daughter and visiting the son at the school. She is hopeful that her son can be able to care for the children eventually and before she dies. She is on thin ice with this process and doesn't want to involve social services right now because she fears her son will lose the kids completely.

When cancer insinuates itself, it is ubiquitous, and bargaining doesn't work. We give to Molly and she gives to us her very best effort, all the while trying to keep the fear monster at bay. We know all her effort is not for herself, but for others and for that she deserves to beat the odds.

PAUL

"This is tough news for me, Doc, and I don't know what to tell my family."

Paul is in today to review a scan that shows diffuse disease. He is alone. Usually I prefer to have family members present when we discuss the staging, but he wanted to see this first. He is trying to control the messaging. He is in his mid-70s, married 50 years with a big family and grandchildren. It's such a surprise to him that there is so much disease, and his eyes fill with tears—but not for himself, for his family. He feels so responsible and that he is letting them down by "getting sick."

He has no pain or symptoms, therefore, if the bright spots on imaging were not there, no one would know (for now). He was telling me that he wants to know, but now I believe he wishes we had not scanned him, perhaps giving him several months before he had to face the drama.

Here's the issue. If we do not know we have a disease, we frequently do not appreciate the time we have. Often people come in and say that they are surprised by how much disease there is or that they "didn't know," but I turn that around and say to them that they were able to live without the burden of cancer, the treatment, and angst for those months or years and that is a good thing, especially if the cancer is not curable. The grieving occurs because perhaps they did not enjoy the time enough. Now that is the sad part. Why do we only come to appreciate life when we know it is fleeting?

For Paul, as difficult as this disease will be to fight, his most challenging dilemma is the family dynamics. He says, "Doc, I am the head of this family.

It's all on me. I am the one who needs to be strong because they will take their cue from my reaction, and I need to control that."

I ask if he intends to share, confide, and plan or bear the burden alone. It is his choice and not mine to force. I will respect his decision, and I am pleased that he wants to prepare them. That is a relief, because often people wishing to protect their families leave them feeling overwhelmed not empowered, devastated not calm, and destitute not enriched. I understand the need to manage the messaging, but I am proud of his courage to face them and prepare for his own future. Making a will, seeing a lawyer, spending time with his close family and seeing other relatives, enjoying the time knowing it is limited. It's actually a gift not appreciated by those of us unaware of the future and a message for us all.

Fannie

"I don't want any of that G… D… Crap!"

I am in for an exciting time since we haven't even met yet, and this hits me as I open the door. Fannie wants to control this meeting, and I am prepared to listen. I ask if she would like to hear more about the disease so we can at least make an educated decision.

"The hell with that! I am not losing my hair. I am not goin' in the hospital. I'm not gonna be a sick old lady."

Frankly, I like the spunk. Now if we could just channel this energy for her benefit. Since we are not going to address the disease, look at scans, or encourage any decisions opposing her, I think we can talk about the radiation, which is what we can do to help her stay out of pain. She is up for that because she does not want any of that "G…D… morphine that makes me like a dope and can't poop for weeks!"

So the radiation and managing constipation is handled. Now the discussion is to help meet her goals at 83 years. She says, "Look, Doc, I'm not trying to be difficult, but I took care of my sick husband with cancer, and the chemo killed him. Then my sister had cancer, and the chemo just about killed her. So I see what happens, and it's no good."

Her aversion to chemotherapy is quite popular, and many people think it is the chemo effects that led to death as opposed to the cancer itself. What they see is the downhill slide. Even if the therapy can keep people well for a time, eventually that time ends if their disease isn't curable. The ultimate effects of the treatment are all the patients and families can remember. **Fannie** is not someone who is going to accept any explanation or influence, and that is fine with me. We decide that once the short course of radiation is done, she will be able to go fishing, which she loves.

She tells me that, "Dyin' is what old people do, so I am not afraid."

Don't we all want to have self-control? Some patients are easily "pushed around," frequently seeing many doctors, going in and out of the hospital, getting procedures and therapy they do not even have a chance to approve. We all do an "informed consent" before any therapy, but really it is overwhelming, often presented as "doctor knows best," and rarely are patients appreciative of the full complicated impact. And so I applaud Fannie and her feistiness. I am excited for a patient taking control and not being controlled. She is a reminder to us all that we are here to help and guide, but the ultimate decision-maker is to be respected always.

BARRY

It's sobering when you are treating more and more people your same age. You witness the chaos for them and for their families and can't help but think about your own "fourth quarter," as my husband likes to call it. While I advise, treat, engage, and support, these events force us to look at our own life and how best to prepare. **Barry's** mom and dad thought they were planning, too. They downsized, minimized, consolidated bank accounts, cleaned out the attic, coordinated doctors, made living wills, emptied closets and sent 50 years of accumulation to charity, dispersed jewelry, catalogued photo albums, and held garage sales. They know, with now limited means, they won't be traveling the world, but their world is mostly family and grandchildren. And so, when their dynamic, robust, fun-loving, and fun-living son is diagnosed with a deadly cancer, they are nothing short of blindsided.

This was not in the preparations for their fourth quarter. There is no organizing and planning for this. Life's greatest stressor, the illness of a child, is heart wrenching, and the death of a child, whatever their age, is devastating. When Barry comes to see me, he is appropriately accompanied by his family. At this point in life, he is most interested in accelerating his career, dating, possibly finding a wife, having fun with his friends, doting on his nieces and nephews, working out, and running marathons. I am not presumptuous to assume I have summarized all of his dreams and activities. He is engaging, handsome, bright-eyed, and quick to smile. He is keeping it together for everyone in the room. The pain and fear is on everyone else's face. If anguish was visible, it is here, thick, mucky, stifling, and all consuming.

As I come through the door, it hits me in the chest, but from the neck up, my eyes go to Barry, I smile and meet his eyes that tell me in a silent blink, "Doc, let's not make a big deal of this, okay?" His need to protect them is as great as theirs to support him. How can we all take a breath? I have to discuss the disease and treatment, and I find a way to dispense with this quickly. They are too numb to have a lot of questions.

The only question generally is, "How long?" But today it is also, "How can this happen to our beautiful son?" There was no way to see this truck coming. It is really, really bad luck (or genes). I can't jolly our way to lift the mood; I can't minimize the hurt. I have to just witness this and agree that it is not okay. Soon the family is weeping, and the son is tear-filled. It is breaking their hearts together. I promise we will do our best and also pray for them all.

Then I come for Barry, and as I walk him to the machine, he softly touches my shoulder and says, "Doc, please help my mom." And now I can't see the hallway as my own tears form.

TINA

"I am the evil twin!"

Petite **Tina** actually seems a little proud of that! I believe she has said that often in her 50 years while her twin brother just rolls his eyes. Tina has a long list of medical problems. She is here with her brother, having been unable to have children and now divorced. With no other family, the "good twin" has his hands full. Tiny Tina is feisty and puts on a good front for her brother. Her cancer diagnosis is manageable but in the background of her "co-morbidities", time will be limited. Tina's brother is a successful business man with a wife and children headed to college. I am happy to see him take time to sit and hold is sister's hand, helping to carry her through this process. He realizes that after years of irritating health problems, surgeries, and drama, this will be her "rate limiting step."

They are not sad, sullen, or worried. It is all very matter-of-fact today. This is another day of "let's just get this done." What moves me are the tender moments, the profound connection. He could answer the questions for her but steps back to allow her power. He is quietly proud of Tina. I am careful here to not overburden. Some family members will give up everything they do if, by helping their loved one, they will impact the success. My role here is to encourage Tim to leave Tina in our care. No need to watch over her treatments, drive her to therapy, catalog every blood test. Just let her have control. This sacred bond I need to respect, but help him choose which activities are important and which are just time suckers. So we come up with a plan that respects Tim's time, Tina's needs, and most importantly helps to cherish this profound relationship. Tim will be here for every important moment, discovery, discussion, and Tina is happy he won't have to "hold her head over the toilet!" We have to find a way for them both to live their individual lives while respecting their joined spirits. We can see that Tina is a lucky lady. They have been together forever, and I am in awe of their combined strength.

THE DOCTORS

"My relatives said, 'Why would anybody choose to go into medicine to be around sick people their whole life, and even harder, cancer patients... what are you thinking?!' Maybe I should have listened to them."

I am hearing this from a young colleague who is overwhelmed today by the pressures of regulation. It's not the patients or the cancers; it's the government requirements for every single thing that we do. It is exhausting and takes us from patient care. Why is there a requirement for an orthopedic surgeon to document every single thing like mammograms, colonoscopies, vaccines, neurology, etc. when a patient with knee arthritis is managed? It's just churning papers, and someone reviewing everything that we do, uninformed in many cases, has to complete a check list. If that patient sees six doctors, instead of them each doing their part, they are all documenting the same things, wasting valuable time and expertise. What a mess. I agree with him that there is much unpleasantness, but none of it is the patient or the patient's fault. We waste our day to get through "peer to peer" discussions for insurers reluctant to give the people back what they paid for—care! I fully sympathize with the doctor this morning.

Soon after, another colleague stops by and shares a similar discussion. People are starting to be worn down and burnt out. My recommendations are the same to both, something I never did at their ages when I was challenged. I tell them to meditate every day, stay away from the news, replenish themselves, and don't expect anyone else to fill them up. As I drive home, I have on Satellite radio and listen to a program with a positive message. Today's is about encouraging ourselves. It is uplifting, empowering, and reminds us to take responsibility for our self-talk. It inspires me, and because I mentioned these messages to both physicians, I smile and hope they are tuned in at that hour.

My experience is that men are far less likely to nourish themselves. I hoped by giving them permission, even just floating the ideas, that they will give it a try. It's selfish on my part. These are two very highly regarded physicians in our field. Patients are fortunate to have their conscientious expertise. We do not want to lose them when it may just take a few minutes a day to "encourage themselves." A good idea for everyone.

DIANE

"What is wrong with women?!"

Diane works and is simultaneously undergoing treatment. Just hop on the table between work projects, and all of that is going well. She is also recovering from a few months of chemo and admits to some fatigue. Unfortunately, one of her female docs is telling her she shouldn't be working. Diane is providing for her family and needs the insurance as well, so she thinks this other doc is completely insensitive to her needs.

"Why make me feel bad? I look great, feel fine, do my job, and try to treat this cancer as a nuisance. Will she take care of me if I lose my insurance?"

Today that's not the only insult. Another woman whispered how tired she looked behind her back, and Diane thought how rude it was to gossip about her while she is trying her best to hold it all together.

"Women are our own worst enemies—present company excluded!" She wears the wig so men don't stare at her bald head; she puts on her clothes and jewelry with panache; she is cheerful and smiling. Today's scowl is unusual, and she just wishes others would buoy her up. It's a week of disgruntlements, and none of it's about the cancer. Interpersonal relationships, even acquaintances, can be so very therapeutic whatever our challenge. I want us to remember to give support.

"*I found myself a cheerleader*" is a great song. Find someone today to cheer. It could be a co-worker, store clerk, super-senior. You may not know that person needs a positive word. I tell Diane about the positive messages app for her phone and give her homework for the next week. I want her to find only the positive messages in life and ignore everything else. Why do we always re-member the negative comments or events more than the positive? I am up for my own "re-braining," as I like to call it, and so I am bringing my associates and patients with me. There is nothing wrong with women. We nurture others but forget to take care of ourselves, and maybe if we do, there will be a well of kindness available for other women.

ELLEN

"I am sick of it! This friggin' pink stuff is everywhere! I can't even get a darn donut without being reminded of breast cancer."

Ellen is referring to the pink-colored powdered sugar on her "Breast Cancer Awareness Month" donut this morning. Since its October, expect to see this everywhere. Like we aren't already aware of it. She is a long-time survivor, but as we know, 1% of women with history of breast cancer have it return per year—making even long term not a cure.

I agree with Ellen. Everyone wants to benefit from the drama of breast cancer, but most patients abhor the pink and some refuse to wear anything that is a reminder. Many are proud of their journey and participate with great passion. Too many companies use the emotionally-charged issue to capitalize on pink products with no donation to any research effort. People are encouraged even at the grocery to donate to breast cancer "charities" without any knowledge of how that money is spent. Too much goes to just supporting big salaries and foundation events with minimum going to anything patient-oriented. I watch the charity navigator to determine where my donations go, and if they aren't giving at least 75% to research, they do not get my money.

My best recommendation, if you are not sure where to donate, is to support your local hospital foundations. That way you know the money stays local and benefits programs where you receive care. In my city, a local personality developed a foundation several years ago, and 100% of the money goes to research at a local medical center. People run, play golf, and have many fundraisers throughout the year. One cancer survivor and a truly national inspiration has found a way to make a real difference. Many genetic testing studies and treatments have evolved from her association with a famous national breast cancer researcher. Their efforts are to be lauded, but the pink sugar covering Ellen's fingers not so much. So I ask her how she intends to honor herself this month.

She says, "You know, Doc, after you told me the story of how you ran your half marathon then called your husband at mile nine and asked for a ride (but instead he encouraged me to finish the race), I thought if you can do it so can I! And so, I am going to run the national breast cancer half marathon here in February! I have been training with the run-walk method and I know I can do it."

What Ellen found was a way to improve her health, stamina, and immune system while supporting her cause—something pink sugar could never do. Thousands come—men and women from across the nation to participate—and I am thrilled that in our own backyard, we can celebrate. Many wear tutus (even the men), pink wigs, and names on their backs of people they are honoring. Whole families take part, some are pushed in wheelchairs, and many run with strollers or with their dogs. It's a joyous event. I will encourage more of my patients to participate—even to do a relay with family will be a wonderful boost when they see all the support. Activities like these are a great refund on your investment. Many volunteer or cheer if they cannot walk or run. It's a real celebration of life, boosting mind, body and all of our spirits!

Irma

Yes, hurricane **Irma**! The pain of destruction first from Harvey and then Irma through the islands, followed by obliteration by Hurricane Maria, is even more shocking when patients are trying to deal with cancer. Pearl, Monica, Jose… so many looking for treatment for cancer while their houses are gone and probably will not return to their former lives. So tragic. They are seeking treatment, first evacuating from St. Thomas to San Juan, now with Maria devastating Puerto Rico, moving again to Florida.

If they have wonderful support, they can make it to us and hope to resume some form of healthcare. There are no buildings or people to call for records. These people are numb. The shock of cancer is now a fleeting memory as basic survival needs must be met. After the flurry of evacuations even here and days without power, those blessed are relieved and recognize our role in helping others pick up the pieces.

A fellow physician has evacuated his entire family from Puerto Rico and has such a wonderful, generous spirit, laughing that he is the only male with eight women in his home! (He may seek evacuation!) I am inspired that he can chuckle with all the drama. Sometimes we can feel so overwhelmed and helpless, but we are not. Every one of us can pitch in and help in some way—support a cause, donate, set up plans to assist. Even the smallest effort is a movement forward. It is a time of coming together for humanity.

It is not the self-absorbed, "I have cancer. What can you do for me? How can I be rescued from this disease?" Today and for the next many months the shift in focus from self to others is occurring not just in the healthcare profession, but in every single person. Look at the lines in Vegas to donate blood after a horror. We truly and deeply want to care for each other. It is what drew me to this profession. Help where you can. Judiciously apply your expertise. Listen to every story. Lend a hand and a kind word. Be patient, kind, gentle, and loving. We may not heal everyone from cancer; we may not rescue everyone from their personal drama. But we can each be a force that joins with others for the greater good.

I hope this window into dialogues has inspired you to listen to your friends and loved ones. I know we are all growing in our outreach and compassion, and I am grateful for the many teachings these patients have provided to help my own awareness. I appreciate the opportunity to share their spirit and amazing courage with you.

We all have stories, and if you have one that you would like to share or see in my next book, please email me at listeningtocancer@yahoo.com

God Bless and Be Well,
Joanne